# THE POCKET DICTIONARY FOR DIALYSIS TECHNICIANS AND NURSES

## 1st Edition

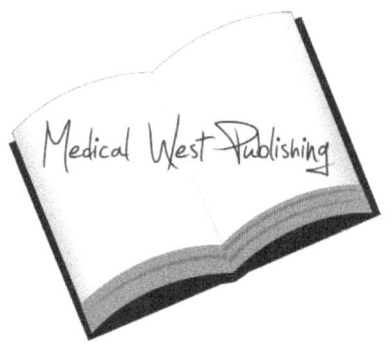

# Medical West Publishing

© Copyright 2012
P.O. Box 22
West Covina, CA. 91793

*All rights reserved. No part of this book may be reproduced in any form or by any means, including information storage and retrieval systems, without permission in writing from the publisher, except by a reviewer who my quote brief passages in a review.*

# THE POCKET DICTIONARY FOR DIALYSIS TECHNICIANS AND NURSES

Oscar M. Cairoli, BSN, MA, RN, PHN

Clinical Director
Renal Business Group
Kaiser Permanente
Pasadena, CA

# Preface

**The Pocket Dictionary for Dialysis Technicians and Nurses** was created to meet a need for the health care giver working in the dialysis field, whether an RN, a LVN/LPN, or a Patient Care Technician.

For the person just entering this complex field, this book provides an organized approach to a very special vocabulary. For the experienced clinician, this book fills the need for quick, on-the-spot reference.

I like to acknowledge the help and support that have been extended to me during the years by dedicated technicians, nurses, physicians, and other members of the renal team. And my deepest appreciation goes to the **dialysis patient** who has giving me the reason to be a nephrology nurse for over 30 years. And last but not least, I like to express my gratitude to Myrna Barrios-Craig for her support during this project.

# TO THE STUDENT/READER

Take this book with you to the clinical area or classes and use it as a reference. **Never stop learning**, to benefit your knowledge base, and ultimate, to benefit our patients.

# DIALYSIS ACRONYMS
# A

# A

**AAMI** – See "Association for the Advancement of Medical Instrumentation"

**ABDOMEN** - The portion of the trunk located between the back, below the diaphragm, and including the lower portion of the abdominopelvic cavity. Contains the stomach, lower part of the esophagus small and large intestines, liver, gallbladder, spleen, pancreas, bladder.

**ABSCESS** – An abscess is a localized infection under the skin that looks like a blister or pimple filled with fluid or pus. If fistula needles are inserted into or near an abscess, infection of the fistula or graft or any other tissues may occur.

**ACCESS** – An access is a route into the blood stream that follows sufficient blood flow for hemodialysis. For a permanent vascular access, a vein is surgically connected to an artery, either directly (arteriovenous fistula) or with a piece of a synthetic tubing called a graft. For a temporary vascular access, a catheter must be inserted into a large central vein, such as the internal jugular vein in the neck. (*See also: Arteriovenous, Fistula, Catheter, and Graft*).

**ACETATE** - A salt of acetic acid.

**ACID** – Acid is a substance with a pH below 7.0 that is capable of donating a hydrogen ion (H+). In the human body, acids are created when protein and other substances are broken down by cell metabolism. Acids are salts, lemon juice, etc. (*See also Buffer, pH*).

**ACIDOSIS** - The hydrogen ion is increased thus the pH is decreased. A pathologic condition esulting from accumulation of acid or depletion of the alkaline reserve in the blood and body tissues.

**ACQUIRED IMMUNODEFFICIENCY SYNDROME (AIDS)** - See Human Immunodeficiency Virus (HIV).

**ACUTE** – Sudden onset. Having severe symptoms and a short course.

**ACUTE RENAL FAILURE** – Acute renal failure (ARF) is kidney failure with a sudden onset. An illness, injury, or toxin that stresses the kidneys usually causes it. In many cases of acute renal failure, patients who survive are able to recover their kidney function with temporary support provided by dialysis. In other cases, patients may develop chronic, irreversible renal failure.

**ADSORB** – To cause particles or molecules in a solution to stick to a surface of a solid material. To attract and retain other material on the surface.

**ADVANCED DIRECTIVES** – Advanced directives are documents that outline a patient's wishes for medical treatment or no treatment (comfort care only), in case the patient becomes too ill to make such decisions at a later date. A living will is an example of an advance directive. The patient's family members and other members of the health care team should be informed of the patient's wishes when an advanced directive has been prepared.

**AIR DETECTOR** – The air detector monitors blood in the venous line of the extra corporeal circuit for air. Air in the patient's blood stream can interfere with blood flow or heartbeat, causing death. If the air detector detects air, an alarm will sound, the blood pump will stop, and the venous bloodline will clamp to prevent air from reaching the patient.

**AIR EMBOLISM** – An air embolism occurs when air bubbles enter the bloodstream and are carried into a vessel small enough to be blocked by the air. In the vessel, the air embolus acts like a clot, blocking the flow of blood. Symptoms depend on the location of the air and the position of the patient. Dialysis machines have monitors to detect air in the venous bloodline to help prevent this potentially fatal complication.

**ALBUMIN** – Albumin is a blood protein that helps regulate osmotic pressure. Low serum albumin levels (<3.5 g/dl) may mean that a patient has malnutrition, which is very common in hemodialysis patients, and is linked to an increase of death. The presence of albumin in the urine indicates malfunction of the kidney, and may accompany kidney disease or heart failure. (*See also: Osmotic Pressure*).

**ALKALOSIS** - A pathologic condition resulting from accumulation of base, or from loss of acid without comparable loss of base in the body fluids.

**ALUM** – An aluminum compound often added to city water supplies to make the water clearer. Aluminum can build up in the bodies of the dialysis patients; therefore, it is important to keep the aluminum in the water used for dialysis at low levels by treating the water used to make dialysate.

**ALUMINUM RELATED BONE DISEASE (ARBD)** – ARBD is a bone disease caused by prolonged exposure to aluminum. Healthy kidneys secrete aluminum as waste. Aluminum builds up in the tissues at the point where new bone forms, can be seen on X-ray. Sources of aluminum include water used for dialysate, medications, and aluminum cookware. Aluminum based phosphate binders are also a source of exposure, but these have widely been replaced with calcium-based binders. The symptoms of ARBD can include deep bone pain, muscle weakness, and possible fractures.

**AMYLOIDOSIS** – Amyloidosis is a disorder thought to result from building-up in the body of a starch-like protein (called beta 2- microglobulin) normally removed by healthy kidneys. This protein is almost insoluble and once it infiltrates the tissues they become waxy and nonfunctioning. The protein is believed to accumulate in the bones, joints, and other tissues of some renal patients, causing arthritis-like joint pain, and/or bone pain. The use of high flux dialysis membrane can remove the beta 2- microglobulin associated with amyloidosis, which may help prevent or treat this disorder.

**ANAPHYLACTIC REACTION** – An anaphylactic reaction, or anaphylaxis, is an immediate severe reaction to a substance to which an individual is allergic. The reaction may include hives, itching, or wheezing; the reaction may develop into anaphylactic shock, causing hypotension, cardiac arrhythmias, or asystole, spasms of breathing passages, and swelling of the throat can even cause death.

**ANASTOMOSIS** – Communication between two vessels. An anastomosis is a surgical connection. In a hemodialysis access, a connection is made between blood vessels – as in a vein and an artery connected to form an arteriovenous fistula. dialysis needles should not be inserted directly into an area of the anastomosis.

**ANATOMY** - The structure of an organism. The branch of science dealing with the form and structure of organisms.

**ANEMIA** – Anemia is a shortage of oxygen-carrying red blood cells. Because red blood cells bring oxygen to all the cells in the body, anemia causes severe fatigue, heart disorders, difficulty concentrating, reduced immune function, and other problems. Anemia is common among renal patients, caused by insufficient erythropoietin, iron deficiency, repeated blood losses, and other factors. Anemia is treated with EPOGEN (Epoitin Alfa), a synthetic form of erythropoietin, and with iron supplements. (*See also: EPOGEN, Erythropoietin, Hematocrit, and Hemoglobin*).

**ANESTHETIC** – An anesthetic is a drug that numbs the body to prevent pain. Local anesthetics can be injected into a certain spot (such as into the skin around a puncture site before needle insertion), or applied to the skin to prevent pain at the site.

**ANEURYSM** – An aneurysm is a ballooning or bulging of a weak spot in a blood vessel. Because the aneurysm can rupture, or burst causing severe bleeding great care must be taken in a patient who has one. Aneurysms can occur if needles are inserted too often into the same area of the fistula.

**ANION** – Ion carrying a negative electric charge.

**ANGIOPLASTY** – Angioplasty is a medical procedure used to dilate, or open up, a narrowed area of a blood vessel, called a stenosis. In dialysis patients, Angioplasty may be used to treat a stenosis in a vascular access. A small balloon is treated through the blood vessel into the access and gently inflated to push the walls of the vessel open.

**ANTEROGRADE** – Anterograde means <u>with the direction</u> of flow. With a fistula or graft, the anterograde flow is the needle pointing away from the anastomosis. (Retrograde means <u>against the flow</u> and the needle tip must be 1 inch away from the anastomosis). The venous needle is always placed anterograde while the arterial needle can be placed anterograde or retrograde in the vascular access.

**ANTICOAGULANT** – A medication or chemical that prevents clotting of the blood. Any substance that in vivo or in vitro suppresses, delays, or nullifies coagulation of the blood. In dialysis patients, anticoagulants, such as heparin, are used to prevent formation of blood clots in the extra corporeal circuit during hemodialysis *(See also: Heparin).*

**ANTIDIURETIC HORMONE (ADH)** – Antidiuretic hormone, or vasopressin, is released by the pituitary gland in the brain. ADH triggers the normal kidneys to reabsorb more water, to help prevent excess fluid loss. Vasopressin also triggers the blood vessels to constrict or tighten.

**ANTISEPTICS** - Antiseptics are products that stop or interfere with the growth of bacteria or viruses. They are used to kill microorganisms, to prevent infection and the spread of disease. *(See also: Microorganisms)*.

**ANTITHROMBOGENIC** - Prevents the formation of clots.

**APICAL PULSE** - The apical pulse is the pulse felt on the chest wall directly over the heart.

**APNEA** - Apnea is the temporary period when breathing stops due to various causes. The prefix "A" before the word means without. Pnea means breathing. In obstructive apnea there is respiratory effort but no air flows because of upper airway obstruction.

**ARRHYTHMIA** - An arrhythmia is an irregularity of the heartbeat, which may be felt as irregular pulses or heard directly over the heart. Also called dsyrythmia. (Without rhythm).

**ARTERIAL PRESSURE** - In dialysis, arterial pressure is measured within the arterial drip chamber, between the patient's arterial needle and the blood pump – as pre-pump arterial pressure. (Can also be measured as post pump pressure – after the blood pump and before the dialyzer).

**ATERIAL PRESSURE MONITOR -** The arterial pressure is measured in the arterial drip chamber and there is a pressure monitor line connected to a transducer protector. The transducer takes the pressure and gives a read out on the monitor (a gauge or screen). The pressure is usually a pre pump blood pressure and is therefore a negative pressure because the blood pump is pulling blood from the patient's vascular access. A positive pressure is when the drip chamber pressure reading is post blood pump. (See *also: Extracorporeal Circuit*).

**ARTERIALIZED -** In creation of an AV fistula, the blood from the artery anastomosed to a vein crosses over, dilates and thickens the vein.

**ARTERIOVENOUS (AV) FISTULA -** A fistula is an opening between body and cavities. In people with renal failure, an arteriovenous fistula is a surgical connection between and artery and a vein. Just beneath the skin of the arm or leg. Dr. James Cimino and Dr. James Brecia developed the surgery in 1966. In an AV fistula, a strong flow of arterial blood is shunted to a vein. The force of the blood flowing from the artery thickens the vein wall. A mature fistula can be punctured repeatedly with dialysis needles and provide the rapid blood flow rates needed for dialysis.

**ARTERY** - An artery is a blood vessel that carries blood away from the heart at high pressure. Arteries deliver oxygenated blood to every part of the body. Arteries have muscles in their walls and veins have valves.

**ARTIFICIAL** – Artificial means man made, usually in imitation of something found in nature. The dialyzer is often called an artificial kidney, because it is a synthetic piece of equipment that imitates the function of a kidney.

**ASCITES** - Ascites is a build up of fluid in the abdomen caused by liver damage, and heart failure, malnutrition or infection. Special ultrafiltration procedures and other methods (i.e. abdominal drainage) may be required to remove the excess fluid.

**ASEPSIS** - Asepsis is the absence of disease producing microorganisms. Asepsis in dialysis is accomplished by disinfection, maintaining dialysis equipment, and using aseptic technique for invasive procedures, such as inserting dialysis needles.

**ASEPTIC** – Aseptic means germ-free, or sterile.

**ASSOCIATION FOR THE ADVANCEMENT OF MEDICAL INSTRUMENTATION** --- Develops voluntary standards for various aspects of dialysis treatment, including maximum levels of water contamination and methods of dialyzer processing.

**AUSCULTATION** – Auscultation means listening with a stethoscope. Auscultation of a patient's vascular access is used to help diagnose problems like stenosis or thrombosis that can change the normal sound of the bruit.

# DIALYSIS ACRONYMS
# B

# B

**BACKFILTRATION** – Back filtration is movement of dialysate across the dialyzer membrane into the patient's blood. It can be caused by a change in the pressure or concentration gradient between dialysate and blood. Backfiltration may be more likely to occur with high flux dialyzer membranes, which have larger pores, and thus are more permeable. Backfiltration can be dangerous to the patient because endotoxins contained in non-sterile dialysate can enter the bloodstream directly causing congestive heart failure. *(See also: Permeable).*

**BACKWASHING** – Backwashing means forcing water backward through a filter. This technique can be used to remove accumulated particles from clogged sediment filters in a water treatment system. *(See also: Filters).*

**BACTERIA** – Plural for bacterium. Bacteria are microscopic, single-cell organisms that can cause disease. Bacteria are classified as gram-positive or gram-negative by the color they turn on a standard laboratory test called Gram's stain. *(See also: Endotoxin, Gram-negative, Gram-positive).*

**BASE** - Base is a chemical that is capable of accepting a hydrogen ion (H+). A substance with a pH of greater than 7.0 is considered to be a base, alkali. In the body, bicarbonate is a base. In the chemical processes of the body, bases are essential to the maintenance of a normal acid-base balance.

**BICARBONATE** - Bicarbonate is a buffer found in the blood that is reabsorbed by health kidneys. Bicarbonate is used by the body to neutralize acids formed when protein and other foods are metabolized. Patients with kidney failure can no longer secrete hydrogen ions and can no longer regulate or reabsorb enough bicarbonate to replenish blood supplies. As a result, these patients cannot neutralize acids very well, so bicarbonate is most commonly used in dialysate to help restore levels of bicarbonate in the body. Bicarbonate buffer has the advantage of being quickly used by the body, making dialysis more comfortable for the patients. The main disadvantage of using bicarbonate dialysate are its ability to support bacterial growth, and the need for two separate dialysate concentrates (acid and bicarbonate) to prevent the formation of precipitate (calcium carbonate or magnesium), that can interfere with the normal operation of dialysis equipment. (*See also: Buffer*).

**BIOCOMPATIBLE** - Means similar to the human body—and thus less likely to cause adverse immune responses normally triggered by a foreign "invader". Some dialyzer membrane materials (such as polysulfone) are considered more biocompatible than cellulose membranes. However cellulose membranes can become more compatible after use. A coating of blood protein develops inside a cellulose dialyzer after it has been used tricking the patient's immune system treating the membrane as less "foreign". (*See also: Cellulose*).

**BLOOD LEAK** – A blood leak occurs when the delicate semipermeable membrane of the dialyzer tears, allowing blood to leak into the dialysate. Severe blood leaks can cause major blood loss during dialysis (Keep in mind that if the blood leaks out, dialysate can enter the bloodstream, which could cause bacteria to enter the patient's blood).

**BLOOD LEAK DETECTOR** – Blood leak detector is an alarm system on the hemodialysis delivery system that monitors used dialysate for blood that would indicate a leak in the dialyzer membrane. Since a triggered alarm would stop the blood pump and the venous line clamps, this is a blood compartment alarm – even though it examines used dialysate. The detector shines a beam of light through the used dialysate into a photocell. Any break in the transmission of the light beam caused by (microscopic) blood cells will trigger the alarm. *(See also: Hemodialysis Delivery System)*.

**BLOOD PATH** - Conduit through which the blood passes. In dialysis, the arterial and venous sets and blood passages within the dialyzer make up a continuous extracorporeal blood path.

**BLOOD PUMP** - The blood pump is the part of the dialysis delivery system that moves the patient's blood through the extracorporeal circuit using a roller pump at a fixed rate of speed. During hemodialysis, the blood tubing is treaded between the pump head and the rollers. The rollers move blood through the extracorporeal circuit and back to the patient.

**BLOOD PRESSURE** - Blood pressure is a measurement of the amount of pressure exerted against the wall of vessels. The systolic blood pressure rises during activity or excitement and falls during sleep. The average blood pressure for a relaxed sitting adult is 120/80. Blood pressure varies with age, sex, altitude, muscular development, and according to states of mental and physical stress and fatigue. The blood pressure is determined by several interrelated factors, including the pumping action of the heart, the resistance to the flow of blood in the arterioles, the elasticity of the walls of the main arteries, the blood volume and extracellular fluid volume, and the blood viscosity, or thickness.

**BLOOD PUMP SEGMENT**- The blood pump segment is durable, larger diameter section of the arterial blood tubing that is threaded through the roller mechanism of the blood pump.

**BLOOD TUBING (OR BLOODLINES)** – Blood tubing is a part of the extracorporeal circuit that transports blood from the patient's vascular access through the arterial puncture site, to and from the dialyzer back to the patient through the venous tubing. There are two segments of blood tubing, the *arterial* (often color-coded red) and *venous* (often color-coded blue). Components of the blood tubing include patient connectors; dialyzer connectors, drip chamber/bubble trap, as well as the blood pump segment, and heparin and saline infusion lines.

**BLOOD UREA NITROGEN** - Urea is a waste product of protein metabolism, measured as blood urea nitrogen (BUN). Because patients with renal failure cannot remove urea from their body, it builds up between treatments and must be removed by dialysis. BUN is easily measured, so it is used as a stand in for other wastes that also build up in the blood between treatments but are difficult to identify. Measurement of BUN is the basis of kinetic modeling and urea reduction ration, methods for determining the adequacy of the dialysis treatment. (*See also: Hemodialysis Adequacy, Urea Kinetic Modeling, Urea Reduction Ratio, and Uremia*).

**BOWMAN'S CAPSULE** - The renal or malpighian corpuscle. It consists of a visceral layer closely applied to the glomerulus and an outer parietal layer. It functions as a filter in the formation of urine.

**BRACHIAL PULSE** - The brachial pulse felt at the brachial artery, in the crease of the elbow. The main artery of the arm.

**BRACHIOCEPHALIC FISTULA** - A brachiocephalic fistula is the most common type of fistula of the upper arm. The fistula is created by surgically joining the brachial artery and the cephalic vein. (*See also: Arteriovenous Fistula*).

**BRUIT** - (French word pronounced brew-ee) A bruit is a swooshing or buzzing sound caused by the high pressure flow of blood through the patient's AV fistula or graft. The bruit can be heard through a stethoscope at the anastomosis, and for some distance along the access. A low pitch bruit with both a systolic and diastolic component indicates a blood flow sufficient to permit dialysis. A high-pitch bruit may indicate stenosis of the access. [Many times a distinctive pulse instead of swooshing sound also indicates clotting of the graft/fistula may occur]. (aneurysmal bruit is a blowing sound heard over an aneurysm).

**BUBBLE TRAP** – See Drip Chamber.

**BUFFER** - A buffer is a substance that maintains the pH of a solution at constant level,
despite the addition of acid or base. Bicarbonate and acetate are two buffers used in dialysis to maintain the pH of dialysate. (*See also: Acid, Bicarbonate).*

**BUN** – See Blood Urea Nitrogen.

**BURETTE** - A graduated glass tube used to deliver a measured amount of liquid.

**BYPASS** – Bypass is a safety feature of the hemodialysis delivery system that cuts off the flow of fresh dialysate to the dialyzer and shunts it to the drain. Bypass prevents unsafe dialysate (wrong conductivity, temperature, or pH) from reaching the patient and causing harm. (*See also: Hemodialysis Delivery System*).

# DIALYSIS ACRONYMS
# C

# C

**CALCITRIOL** – Calcitriol is the activated form of Vitamin D, produced by healthy kidneys, which is needed by the body to absorb calcium from food. Many dialysis patients need calcitriol supplements to turn off the PTH and to help avoid secondary hyperparathyroidism and bone disease. (*See also: Secondary Hyperthyroidism*).

**CALCIUM** – Calcium is an element that exists as a cation (positively charged ion) that is partly bond to protein in the blood. In the human body, calcium is an electrolyte needed for nerve and muscle function and normal bone formation. Too much or too little calcium in dialysate feed water supply can cause serious complications for the patients, including death. Calcium in a dialysis feed water supply can combine with other substances to form precipitate or scale that can clog dialysis machinery if bicarbonate buffered dialysate is used. Patient blood levels of calcium are usually checked monthly. (*See also: Electrolyte, Hypercalcemia, and Hypocalcemia*).

**CANNULA** - A tube that is inserted into an opening in the body. See: Shunt.

**CAPD** – See Continuous Ambulatory Peritoneal Dialysis.

**CAPILLARIES** - Capillaries are the body's smallest blood vessels, where blood crosses arteries to veins. Capillaries are even smaller in diameter that human hair; blood cells must line up single file to pass through. Unlike arteries and veins, capillary walls are semipermeable, allowing oxygen, food, and waste products to pass through. In the kidneys the glomerulus is a tiny ball of capillaries that filters out wastes, small essential solutes, and water from the blood because they are small enough to go through the selective glomerular membrane.

**CARBON TANK** – Carbon tanks are water treatment devices that contain granular activated carbon that absorbs molecular weight particles from water. Carbon tanks are used primarily to remove chlorine, chloramines, pesticides, and some trace organic substances from water used in dialysis.

**CARDIAC ARREST** – Cardiac arrest is a situation which the heart stops beating. Cardiac arrest can be a lethal side effect of certain dialysis incidents, such as the use of too warm dialysate, improper dialysate concentration, hemolysis, loss of too much blood, or a large amount of air entering the patient's blood stream. Hyperkalemia also can cause cardiac arrest. Synonyms that you need to know: asystole (without heartbeat), cardiac standstill, flat line (*See Also: Hemolysis and Hyperkalemia*).

**CARDIAC OUTPUT** - Cardiac output is the amount of blood passing through the heart in a certain period of time. The presence of an AV fistula or graft causes a 10% increase in the size of the heart. Patients who cannot tolerate this change in cardiac output are not good candidates for AV fistulae or grafts. (*See also: Arteriovenous Fistula*).

**CARDIAC TAMPONADE** - Cardiac Tamponade is a condition resulting from pericarditis (an accumulation of fluid in the pericardial sac) where the heart cannot beat accurately due to the fluid in the pericardial sac.

**CARPAL TUNNEL SYNDROME** - Paresthesias, pain, or numbness affecting some part of the median nerve distribution of the hand(s), i.e., palmar side of thumb, index finger, and radial half of the ring finger, and radial half of the palm. The parethesias and pain may radiate into the arm. There may be a history of cumulative trauma to the wrist, e.g., in carpenters, rowers, or those who regularly use vibrating tools or machinery.

**CAPILLARY FLOW** - A term used to describe a type of parallel-flow dialyzer in which the blood flows through tiny capillary-like tubes made of a semipermeable membrane. The mechanism by which a liquid rises in small tubes or fibers.

**CATABOLISM** – Catabolism is a complex chemical process in which substances (e.g., proteins) are broken down into simpler substances in the blood, producing waste products. The opposite of anabolism. Healthy kidneys normally remove these wastes (e.g. urea), but in dialysis patients, it must be removed during dialysis treatment.

**CATHETER** - A catheter is a plastic tube. In hemodialysis, a catheter is used to create a temporary or longer-term dialysis access. Catheters are often temporary or permanently implanted into the internal jugular vein (neck), femoral vein (groin), or subclavian vein (chest). The internal jugular and femoral sites are less likely than subclavian sites to cause central venous stenosis, a complication that can reduce the number of potential access sites the patient has. For this reason, NKF-DOQI guidelines recommend use of the internal jugular for hemodialysis catheters, when possible. In peritoneal dialysis, a catheter is surgically placed in the abdomen to allow fresh dialysate to be infused into the peritoneal cavity and used dialysate to be drained. (*See also: Central Venous Stenosis, Peritoneal Dialysis*).

**CATION** - A cation is a positively charged ion. In water treatment, cations can be removed by ion exchange or reverse osmosis water treatment to ensure acceptable contents of water used for dialysate and reprocessing. (*See also: Deionizer, Ion*).

**CCPD** – See continuous Cycling Peritoneal Dialysis.

**CELL** - A mass of protoplasm containing a nucleus or nucleal material. It is the unit of structure of all animals and plants. The basic structural unit of living organisms. All living cells arise from other cells, either by division or by fusion.

**CELLULOSE** – Cellulose is a fiber that forms the cell walls of plants. Cellulose acetate was the first material used as a dialyzer membrane by Dr. Willem Kolff in 1942. In water treatment, cellulose acetate was also the first material used to form reverse osmosis membranes. To form a membrane, cellulose can be dissolved in a solution containing copper salts and ammonium. The resulting material is formed into sheet of hollow fibers using a solution-spinning technique. Cellulose dialyzer membranes are the most likely to cause first-use syndrome in some patients, because of this they are not considered biocompatible. (*See also: Biocompatible, First-Use Syndrome*).

**CENTRAL VENOUS STENOSIS** - Central venous stenosis is a narrowing of the central veins of the body that can make the arm on the affected side of unsuitable for a vascular access. With a limited number of potential vascular access sites available in the human body, it is important to preserve as many as possible. High rates of central venous stenosis are the reason that the subclavian vein is not recommended by the NKF-DOQI guidelines for hemodialysis catheter placement.

**CFU** - See colony forming units.

**CHLORAMINES** - Chloramines are substances formed by mixing chlorine and ammonia, or created in nature when chlorine combines with organic material. Ammonia is added to municipal water supplies to boost the germ killing power of chlorine. Chlorine is an oxidant, a substance that destroys microorganisms by breaking their cell walls. If chloramines contaminate dialysis water, they can cause a serious condition called hemolysis (rupture of red blood cells) in patients. Carbon tanks are used to remove chloramines from water use for dialysis. (*See also: Carbon Tank*).

**CHLORIDE** – Chloride is a salt concentrate needed in dialysate and in the human body. Chloride combines with other elements to form sodium chloride, potassium chloride, magnesium chloride, and calcium chloride.

**CHLORINE** - The element chlorine is a greenish-yellow gas that can cause severe irritation to the lungs if inhaled. Chlorine is combined with other ingredients (such as in sodium hypochlorite-bleach) to disinfect surfaces. Chlorine may also be added to the municipal water supplies to destroy microorganisms. Carbon tanks are used to remove chlorine and chloramines from water used for hemodialysis and the dialyzer reuse.

**CHRONIC RENAL FAILURE (CRF) -** Chronic means ongoing, continuing, or long-term. Chronic renal failure is a long, usually slow process that involves progressive loss of nephrons, and thus loss of kidney function. Chronic renal failure can take many years and may not cause symptoms until advanced stage. End-stage renal disease (ESRD) is an endpoint of chronic renal failure; if refers to the point at which renal replacement therapy (e.g. dialysis) is required for survival. (*See also: End Stage Renal Disease, Nephrons*).

**CLEARANCE (K) -** Clearance is a quantity of blood (in ml) that is completely cleared of a solute in one minute of dialysis at a given blood flow rate and dialysate rate.
Clearance is a measure of dialyzer performance, and is one of the characteristics of dialyzers that can affect the dialysis effectiveness. Manufactures often test dialyzers with solutions other than blood (in vitro), so actual clearance of a given dialyzer during dialysis (in vivo) can vary significantly from the manufacturer's stated clearance. Mathematical expression of the rate at which a given substance is removed from a solution. (*See also: Hemodialysis Adequacy*).

**CLINICAL PRACTICE GUIDELINES -** Clinical practice guidelines are recommendations for patient care developed by expert panels and/or by a thorough review of medical literature. The National Kidney Foundation-Dialysis Outcomes Quality Initiative (NKF-DOQI) guidelines released in 1997 cover four key areas of Nephrology: Anemia, hemodialysis adequacy, peritoneal dialysis adequacy, and vascular access. The goal of the NKF-DOQI clinical practice guidelines is to improve patient outcomes. (*See also: Patient Outcomes*).

**COEFFICIENT OF ULTRAFILTRATION (KUF)** - The kuf is the fixed amount of fluid that a dialyzer will remove from the patient's blood per hour, at a specified pressure. The kuf is also called the ultrafiltration factor (UFF) or ultrafiltration rate (UFR) and is expressed in milliliters (ml) per hour (hr) of water removed for each millimeter (mm) of mercury (hg) of transmembrane pressure (TMP), or ml/hr/mm/Hg TMP. The higher the KUF, the more fluid per millimeter of mercury pressure will be removed. High-flux and high-efficiency dialyzers have higher kuf's than conventional dialyzers. Any KUF above 8 requires the use of volumetric control hemodialysis systems to precisely control the amount of fluid removed.

**COLONY FORMING UNITS**- The number of colony forming units (CFU) in a water or dialysate unit is measured by the number of living (able to form colonies) bacteria.

**COMPOSITE RATE REIMBURSEMENT SYSTEM** - A composite rate reimbursement system is a method of U.S Government payment for dialysis treatment. Dialysis facilities are paid a fixed, limited amount of money for each dialysis treatment given to a patient. The limited amount, the composite rate, must cover nearly all the services to dialysis patients.

**CONCENTRATION** - Concentration is the amount of solute(s) (i.e., potassium, sodium) dissolved in a measured amount of fluid (i.e., water, blood) A highly concentrated solution had more solutes and less fluid. The urine is concentrated, so that the proper amounts of fluid and other substances are retained in the body. In dialysis, the concentration of each of the substances in dialysate must be correct, to ensure a safe and effective procedure.

**CONCENTRATON GRADIENT** - See Gradient.

**CONDUCTIVE SOLUTE TRANSFER** - See diffusion.

**CONDUCTIVITY** - Conductivity is the ability of a solution to conduct electricity. It is a measure of ions in solution. A conductivity meter measures the electrolyte composition (or how many ions in a solution) of dialysate by measuring the dialysate's ability to conduct an electrical current; to be sure it is within the safe limit. Capacity for conductance.

**CONDUCTIVITY ALARM** – The conductivity alarm indicates an inappropriate mixture of water and dialysate concentrate. If this alarm has triggered, the dialysis machine will go into bypass mode, shunting dialysate to the drain.

**CONFIDENTIALITY** - Confidentiality is maintaining patient privacy. Patient information should be shared with the rest of the dialysis team when it is medically necessary. Patient information should not be shared outside the dialysis facility, or with other patients or visitors within or outside the facility.

**CONGESTIVE HEART FAILURE (CHF)** - Congestive heart failure occurs when the heart cannot pump out all the blood it receives, so that excess fluid backs up into the lungs. Fluid overload caused by too much fluid intake or not removing enough fluid during dialysis can lead to congestive heart failure. S/S: SOB/dyspnea and +4 leg/ankle/foot edema, have the patient turn their head to the side and look for distended neck veins.

**CONTAMINATE** - Substance or organisms that stains or soils and makes unfit for use.

**CONTINUOUS AMBULATORY PERITONEAL DIALYSIS (CAPD) -** CAPD is a form of peritoneal dialysis that can be done while the patient does his or her usual daily activities. Dialysate enters the patient's peritoneum through a catheter. The dialysate is allowed to remain in the patient's abdomen for a period of time (dwell), and then fresh dialysate is exchanged for used dialysate. Usually four to five exchanges are performed each day. Because dialysis occurs continuously, the patient's blood does not build up large amounts of wastes between treatments; the diet and fluids are less restricted that for hemodialysis patients. (*See also: Peritoneal Dialysis*).

**CONTINUOUS CYCLING PERITONEAL DIALYSIS (CCPD) -** CCPD can be learned after the patient has mastered CAPD. CCPD uses a machine "cycler" to put fluid into the patient's abdomen and drain in out at prescribed periods of time. The process is repeated with fresh dialysate for 8 too 12 hours, usually while the patient sleeps. The last exchange must be left in the abdomen, so the patient can continue to dialyze all day. (*See also: Peritoneal Dialysis*).

**CONTINUOUS QUALITY IMPROVEMENT-** CQI is a management theory based on the idea of constant improvement beyond the status quo. To be successful, all employees and administrators must use a philosophy of constant improvement. CQI often includes a cycle of planning procedures, implementing them, and checking performance (Plan-Do-Check-Act). In dialysis CQI can be a powerful tool for improving patient care.

**CONTINUOUS RENAL REPLACEMENT THERAPY (CRRT) -**
CRRT is a form of extracorporeal therapy that uses either the patient's own heart or a pump to remove blood through an extracorporeal circuit. Usually CRRT is done continuously over many hours to very gently remove extra fluid and some wastes in patients to ill or too unstable for regular hemodialysis (usually in ICU) A cartridge containing a semipermeable membrane (Similar to a hemodialyzer is used).

**CONFECTION, CONVECTIVE SOLUTE TRANSFER -** See solute drag.

**CONVENTIONAL DIALYSIS -**
Conventional dialysis uses a dialyzer with an invitro KUF below 6 to remove wastes and excess fluid from the patients with renal failure. Conventional dialysis treatments often take between 4 and 5 hours to achieve adequate dialysis. (*See also: Coefficient or Ultrafiltration, In Vivo*).

**CUPRAMMONIUM PROCESS -**
Technique for producing regenerated

cuprammonium cellulose membrane using an ammoniacal copper solution.

**COUNTERCURRENT FLOW** - A countercurrent flow within a dialyzer occurs when blood moves in one direction and dialysate flows in the opposite direction during dialysis. Countercurrent flow allows for the most efficient dialysis, because it keeps the blood in constant contact with fresh dialysate. Also known as flow geometry.

**CREATININE** - Creatinine is a waste product of creatinine and creatinine phosphate,
an energy-storing molecule in the muscles normally excreted in urine. Creatinine is produced in proportion to muscle mass, that is, larger people with more muscle mass have higher creatinine levels. Since creatinine is normally produced in fairly constant amounts as a result of the breakdown of phosphocreatine and is excreted in the urine, an elevation in the creatinine level in the blood indicates a disturbance in kidney function.

**CREATININE CLEARANCE** - Creatinine clearance is a urine test that measures the kidney's ability to remove creatinine and other wastes from the blood. As chronic renal failure progresses, creatinine clearance will fall to 10% of normal or less. (*See also: Chronic Renal Failure*).

**CRENATION** - Crenation is a shriveling of blood cell that occurs if the blood cells are exposed to a solution more concentrated than blood. For example, crenation may occur if dialysate with too much concentrate and not enough water is used (hypertonic solution) if crenation occurs, the blood will appear dark red. The condition can be fatal.

**CUFFED-TUNNELED CATHETERS -** Cuffed tunneled catheters are permanent dialysis catheters that are inserted into a blood vessel through a tunnel created under the patient's skin. Inside the tunnel tract, surround tissue grows into an attached cuff to help stabilize the catheter and provide a physical barrier to bacteria.

**CYANOSIS -** Cyanosis is the condition of having bluish-colored skin, lips, gums, and fingernail beds due to lack of oxygen. This condition may be present in patients with fluid overload that have no yet reached congestive heart failure stage. This condition also accompanies methemoglobinemia, caused by exposure to dialysate water contaminated with nitrates.

**CYANOTIC -** The nature of an affected area to turn blue due to the lack of oxygen.

**CYTOLOGY -** The science that deals with the formation, the structure, and the function of cells.

# DIALYSIS ACRONYMS
# D

# D

**DALTON** - The molecular weight or average weight of a molecule (solute) that is measured in Daltons. (Dialyzers can be selected to remove solutes ranging in size from 3,000 Daltons to more than 15,000 daltons).

**DEHYDRATION** - Dehydration is a condition that occurs when the body does not have enough water. If dehydration occurs, due to repeated diarrhea, vomiting, excess sweating or excess fluid removal during dialysis, the patient may have low blood pressure, sunken eyes, listlessness (lack of interest in surroundings), and poor skin tugor (tone). *(See also: Hypotension)*.

**DEIONIZER** - A deionizer is a component of a water treatment system that uses beds of resin beads to remove unwanted ions from water. The dionizer may have one bed to remove cations and a second bed of anions, and a third; mixed bed to remove all ions. The unwanted ions are exchanged for hydrogen (H+) and hydroxide (OH-) ions from water (H2O). *(See also: Cation, Ion)*.

**DELIVERY SYSTEM** - Mechanism for producing properly mixed dialyzing solution from dialysis concentrate and treated water and delivering it to the artificial kidney at a temperature of 37 ° C. *(See also Hemodialysis Delivery System)*.

**DIABETES MELLITUS -** A chronic disorder of carbohydrate metabolism, characterized by hyperglycemia and glycosuria and resulting from inadequate production or utilization of insulin. Persons fulfilling these conditions are not a homogenous group. Diabetes Mellitus is classified according to two syndromes: Type I, or insulin-dependent diabetes mellitus (IDDM) and type II, or non-insulin dependent diabetes mellitus (NIDDM).

**DIABETIC NEPHROPATHY -** Diabetic Nephropathy is kidney disease that occurs as a result of diabetes. Diabetes, a failure of the body to utilize glucose (sugar), is the leading cause of renal failure in the U.S. Diabetes also causes damage to the small arteries in the body, which supply blood to the eyes, kidneys, nervous system, and gastrointestinal system.

**DIALYSATE -** Dialysate is a mixture of treated water and carefully measured chemical that is used to clean the patient's blood during dialysis. Substance such as sodium, calcium, magnesium, chloride, potassium, glucose, and bicarbonate are usually present in the dialysate, in concentrations, similar to normal blood. These concentrations must be very precise, and the dialysate must be mixed properly, or patients can be harmed. In hemodialysis, a semi permeable membrane separates blood and dialysate. Wastes in the blood diffuse across the membrane and into the dialysate, while needed substances diffuse into the blood from the dialysate. In peritoneal dialysis, blood and dialysate are separated by the peritoneum, which acts like a semipermeable membrane. (*See also: Hemodialysis, Osmosis, And Semipermeable Membrane*).

**DIALYSATE DELIVERY SYSTEM** - See Hemodialysis Delivery System.

**DIALYSATE PATH** - Conduit through which the dialyzing solution and dialysate pass.

**DIALYSIS** - Dialysis is a process of removing wastes and excess fluid from the body that damaged kidneys can no longer remove. To maximize the patient's health, the physician will usually prescribe a special renal diet, medications, and other treatments that serve as a supplement to dialysis therapy. Dialysis may be performed using an artificial kidney or dialyzer (hemodialysis) or the patient's own peritoneum (peritoneal dialysis). A dialyzer (containing a semipermeable membrane), dialysate and delivery system are needed to perform hemodialysis. (*See also: Dialysate, Hemodialysis, Hemodialysis Delivery System, Peritoneal Dialysis, and Semipermeable Membrane*).

**DIALYSIS ACIDOSIS** - Metabolic acidosis due to prolonged hemodialysis in which the pH of the dialysis bath has been inadvertently reduced by the action of contaminating bacteria.

**DIALYSIS CHAIN** - A dialysis chain is a corporation that owns many facilities, often in different parts of the country. Each year, the larger chains grow in size independent, hospital-based, and smaller chains are incorporated into the larger chains.

**DIALYSIS DEMENTIA** - See Encephalopathy.

**DIALYSIS DISEQUILIBRIUM SYNDROME** - Dialysis disequilibrium syndrome is a condition in which rapid or drastic changes in the patient's extracellular fluid affect the brain. Urea transfers more slowly from the brain tissue to the blood, so fluid is drawn into the brain, causing swelling. Dialysis disequilibrium syndrome occurs most often in acute renal failure, or when BUN values are very high. (*See also: Blood Urea Nitrogen*).

**DIALYSIS PRINCIPLES** - Dialysis principles are basic scientific processes that make dialysis possible: flow, pressure, resistance, solute transfer (primarily by diffusion), filtration, diffusion and osmosis. The dialysis principles help us to understand what happens within the body, the dialyzer, and the delivery system during the process of dialysis therapy. (*See also: Filtration, Flow, Osmosis, Pressure, and Resistance*).

**DIALYZER** - The dialyzer, or hemodialyzer (also known as the artificial kidney), is a manufactured semipermeable membrane encased in plastic support structure. Dialyzers are used in hemodialysis to remove wastes and fluid from the blood of patients with kidney failure. The semipermeable membrane keeps blood and dialysate separate but allows an exchange of certain solutes and fluids to occur. (*See also: Hollow Fiber Dialyzer, Semipermeable Membrane*).

**DIALYZER REPROCESSING** - See reprocessing, reuse.

**DIALYZING SOLUTION** - A properly mixed isotonic solution that is on the opposite site of the membrane from blood in the dialyzer. It is used to set up a concentration gradient within the artificial kidney.

**DIASTOLIC** - Diastolic pressure is the least pressure of blood against the arteries when the heart is at rest (or between beats). It is the bottom number of a blood pressure reading. *(See also: Systolic)*.

**DIFFUSION** - Diffusion is a scientific principle meaning: dissolved solutes/particles will move form an area of greater concentration to an area of lesser concentration across a semipermeable membrane until the concentration of solutes/particles are equal on both sides of the membrane. In dialysis, diffusion works to remove excess solutes/particles (i.e. waste products) from the blood. Because dialysate is formulated with no wastes (BUN and creatinine), wastes in the blood diffuse across the membrane into the dialysate. The speed of diffusion depends on many factors, such as concentration difference between fluids (concentration gradient), the temperature of dialysate, the size of pores in the semipermeable membrane, and the size of particles. Diffusion is also called conductive solute transport.

**DISEQUILIBRIUM SYNDROME** - See Dialysis Disequilibrium Syndrome.

**DISINFECTION** - The process of disinfecting a surface or material with a disinfectant to inhibit the growth of harmful microbes.

**DISINFECTANT** - A disinfectant is a substance used to destroy or inhibit the growth of microbes. Disinfectant require time to act, and must remain moist and in contact with a surface to be effective. Commonly used for dialysis equipment include formaldehyde, bleach, and gluteraldehye. Commonly used disinfectants for dialyzer reprocessing equipment include formaldehyde, renalin, gluteraldehyde, citric acid, and amuchina. Other uses for disinfectants in dialysis includes cleaning ports on components of the water treatment system before taking a water sample, and wiping off surfaces in the dialysis facilities. (Hibicleans, and Betadine are favorites.)

**DISTAL** - Distal means far. In anatomy, distal is far from the center of the body. The hands and feet are distal extremities.

**DISTAL CONVOLUTED TUBULE** - The distal convoluted tubule is located in the kidney, which lies between the Loop of Henle and the collecting duct. (*See also*: *Ilius*).

**DIURESIS** - Increased output of urine.

**DIURETIC** - A diuretic is a medication that increases the amount of urine produced. The use of certain diuretics can lead to hypokalemia because they promote the loss of potassium in urine. Diuretics are used for patient's pre-ESRD, or prior to starting dialysis. (*See also: Hypokalemia*).

**DOCUMENTATION** - Documentation is a recording of information regarding the patient's care into the permanent medical record or chart. Documentation is important to track the patient's progress, provide a means to follow up each patient's response to treatment, and ensure continuity of care. A patient's medical record provides legal evidence of the care the patient received. Units have specific policies and procedures for documenting patient care.

**DORSAL CAVITY** - The body cavity that is located toward the back (posterior) of the body, it is divided into the cranial cavity which contains the brain and the vertebral cavity, which contains the spinal cord.

**DRIP CHAMBER / BUBBLE TRAP -** An arterial or venous drip chamber reflects arterial or venous pressure in the extracorporeal circuit, using a monitoring line. A bubble trap inside the drip chamber collects any air that may have accidentally entered the blood tubing.

**DRY ULTRAFILTRATION -** See isolated ultrafiltration (DUF, IUF, PUF).

**DRY WEIGHT -** A person with renal failure is said to be at a "dry weight" if there are no signs of fluid overload or dehydration, respiration is normal—with out evidence of fluid in the lungs— and the blood pressure is normal for the patient, neither too high nor too low. "Target weight" is the goal weight for a particular dialysis treatment, and is usually determined by the dry weight.

**DWELL TIME -** In hemodialysis, dwell time is the length of time a disinfectant needs to stay in a dialyzer long enough to ensure proper disinfection during reprocessing. Also for hemodialysis delivery system disinfection, if a chemical disinfectant is used, it must dwell in the delivery system fluid pathways long enough to kill bacteria, and then thoroughly rinse. In peritoneal dialysis, dwell time is the length of time dialysate remains inside the patient's abdomen before it is drained out and replaced with fresh dialysate. (*See also: Reprocessing*).

**DYSPNEA** - Dyspnea mean trouble breathing, or shortness of breath. Dyspnea can be a symptom of anemia, fluid overload, lung or heart problems, or other dialysis complications such as air embolism (air entering the bloodstream). (*See also: Air Embolism, Anemia, Pulmonary Edema, and Uremia*).

# DIALYSIS ACRONYMS
# E

# E

**ECCHYMOSIS** - An ecchymosis is a bruise or bleeding under the skin, causing skin discoloration. In dialysis patients, ecchymosis can be a sign that too much heparin has been administered or that inadequate pressure was placed on the needle site after the needles were removed.

**EDEMA** - Edema is water retention/swelling in the body tissues that occurs as a result of fluid overload or other conditions. The swelling may be observed in the patient's eyelids, ankles, feet, hands, abdomen, or lower back area. "Pitting" edema is when a finger is pushed against the skin of the ankles and leaving a dent. This condition should be reported to a nurse (If it is new for that patient). (*See also: Dry weight, Pulmonary Edema*).

**EFFERENT ARTERIOLE** - A small artery that carries blood away from the glomeruli of the kidney.

**ELECTROLYTE** - An electrolyte is a compound (such as sodium, potassium, and calcium) that breaks apart into ions (electrically charged particles) when dissolved in water. Electrolytes transport electrical impulses along the nerves to the muscles, including the heart. In the body, healthy kidneys maintain electrolyte balance. Electrolytes are added to the dialysate in carefully controlled amounts. Also called ions and can be positive or negative charged particles.

**EMBOLUS** – A mass of undissolved matter present in a blood vessel, which may be solid, liquid or gaseous. Emboli can cause occlusion or blockage of the vessel. (*See also:* A*ir Embolism*).

**EMPTY BED CONTACT TIME -** Empty bed contact time is the time period during which the feed water must remain in contact with the charcoal bed in a carbon tank during water treatment. Feed water must remain in contact with the charcoal long enough to allow adequate removal of chlorine and chloramines. (*See also: Carbon Tank, Chloramines, and Feed Water*).

**ENCEPHALOPATHY -** Encephalopathy is a defect in the function of brain tissues that can be fatal. The symptoms include confusion, short-term memory problems, personality changes, speech problems, muscle spasms, hallucinations, seizure and intellectual impairment. One cause of encephalopathy is chronic exposure to high levels of aluminum in dialysis water. Sources of aluminum include dialysate water, antacids, laxatives, and cookware.

**ENDOCARDIUM -** Serous lining membrane of inner surface and cavities of the heart. It is continuous with the intimae or the interior coat of arteries.

**ENDOCRINE FUNCTION** - Endocrine function, the production of hormones, is one of the tasks of healthy kidneys. Kidneys manufacture hormones that adjust blood pressure (angiotensin) and stimulate red blood cells formation (erythropoietin). Healthy kidneys also convert vitamin D into an activated for that the body can use to absorb calcium to maintain healthy bones (Calcitriol). (*See also: Hormones*).

**ENDOTOXIN** - Endotoxins (lippopolysaccharide) is a toxic component that forms part of the cell walls of bacteria. Licing bacteria can shed endotoxin, and endotoxins are also released when bacteria die and decompose. Because endotoxins are <u>not alive</u>, disinfectants cannot kill it. However, if endotoxin is allowed to enter the patient's body, it can cause pyrogenic (fever) reactions. Endotoxin is a concern in water treatment and dialyzer reprocessing; numbers are decreased by reducing the numbers of bacteria in the water or by using an ultrafilter to remove endotoxin. (*See also: Pyrogenic Reaction, Ultrafilter*).

**END-STAGE RENAL DISEASE (ESRD)**
- ESRD is a legal term for complete and irreversible loss of kidney function, the last stage of chronic renal failure, when renal replacement therapy must be started if the patient is to live. Patients are generally considered to have ESRD when the glomerular filtration rate has dropped to about 10%

of normal. (5 to 10 ml/min). (*See also: Chronic Renal Failure, Glomerular Filtration Rate*).

**EPICARDIUM -** The inner visceral layer of the pericardium, which forms a serous membrane, forming the outermost layer of the wall of the heart.

**EPOGEN (EPOETIN ALFA) -** Epogen is a recombinant (cloned) form of erythropoietin, a hormone that stimulates the bone morrow to form red blood cells.
EPOGEN injected intravenously (into a vein) or subcutaneously (into the tissue beneath the skin), is used to treat anemia of chronic renal failure, eliminating the need for most blood transfusions in dialysis patients and improving their quality of life. Common side effects include hypertension and flu-like symptoms. (*See also: Anemia, Erythropoietin, and Recombinant*).

**EQUILIBRIUM -** Equilibrium is the state of balance. Diffusion (the movement of solutes) occurs until there is an equal concentration on both sides of a semipermeable membrane-until equilibrium has been reached. (*See also: Diffusion, Osmosis, and Semipermeable Membrane*).

**ERYTHROCYTE -** A mature red blood cell or corpuscle. The body of the cell consists of a sponge-like stroma containing a respiratory pigment, hemoglobin, enclosed in a cell membrane of proteins in combination with lipoid substances.

**ERYTHROPOIETIN (EPO)** - Erythropoietin is a hormone produced by healthy kidneys that stimulates bone marrow to produce red blood cells. Anemia caused by using EPOGEN can now treat a shortage of erythropoietin in dialysis patients. Epotin Alfa is a synthetic form of erythropoietin. (*See also: Anemia*).

**ESRD** - See End Stage Renal Disease.

**ESRD NETWORKS** - The ESRD networks were established by the U.S government in 1978 to oversee dialysis facilities and ensure that patients receive high quality care. The networks collect data, implement quality improvement, encourage rehabilitation, establish a grievance procedure for patients, and provide resource materials to ESRD for staff and patients.

**EHTYLENE OXIDE (ETO)** - ETO is a gas used by some manufacturers to sterilize new dialyzers. Patients who are hypersensitive to ETO may suffer the effects of first use syndrome if a new dialyzer that has been sterilized with ETO is not properly rinsed. (ETO is ethylene oxide). (*See also: First Use Syndrome, Hypersensitivity*).

**EXCRETORY FUNCTION** -To excrete means to eliminate from the body. An important excretory function of healthy kidneys it is to rid the body of wastes and excess fluid by producing urine.

Urine contains excess body water and a high concentration of waste products.

**EXSANGUINATION** - Exsanguination is the severe loss of blood that may be life threatening. Common preventable causes of exsanguinations include needle dislodgment, bloodline separation, access rupture, or cracked dialyzer casing.

**EXTRACELLULAR** - Extracellular means outside the cells or surrounding the tissue and also includes the interstitial and intravascular compartments. Extracellular fluid makes up about 1/3 of all the fluid in the body at any given time. Of this fluid about 2/3 is found between organ tissues (interstitial), and the rest is the vascular space (blood vessels), to be removed by dialysis. The sodium level in the dialysate helps ensure the movement of fluid from one fluid compartment to the other.

**EXTRACELLULAR FLUID** - Tissue fluid or fluid occupying spaces between the spaces of cells.

**EXTRACORPOREAL** - Extracorporeal means outside of the body. Hemodialysis is extracorporeal therapy, because it takes place outside the body.

**EXTRACORPOREAL CIRCUIT** - The extracorporeal circuit is an extension of the patient's blood vessels outside of the body. The circuit carries the patient's blood from the access to the dialyzer, and back to the patient. Components of the extracorporeal circuit include the arterial bloodline, dialyzer, venous bloodline, and extracorporeal circuit monitors. *(See also: Blood Tubing, Dialyzer)*.

**EXTRACORPOREAL CIRCUIT MONITORS** - The extra corporeal circuit monitors include blood flow monitor, arterial or venous pressure monitors (measured at the drip chambers), an air detector, and a blood leak detector. These monitors shut off the blood pump and clamp the venous bloodline when the present limits are exceeded on the arterial and venous bloodline, or when blood is detected in the spent dialysate by the blood leak detector. *(See also: Air Detector, Arterial Pressure, Blood Leak Detector, and Venous Pressure)*.

**EXTRACORPOREAL SYSTEM** - The venous and arterial bloodlines that includes the dialyzer for the hemodialysis machine. *(See also: Extracorporeal Circuit)*.

**EXTRASKELETAL CALCIFICATION** - Extraskeletal calcification is the depositing of crystals of calcium phosphate in the patient's blood vessels or soft tissues. The condition can potentially cause gangrene. Hypercalcemia with hyperphosphatemia can cause extraskeletal calcification. Mottled, painful, purplish skin is a symptom of extraskeletal calcification that should be reported immediately to the nurse or nephrologist. (*See also: Hypercalcemia, Hyperphosphatemia*).

# DIALYSIS ACRONYMS
# F

# F

**FEED WATER** - Feed water is untreated tap water before it passes through a water treatment system. Feed water must pass through the various components of a water treatment system before being used for dialysis.

**FEMORAL CATHETER** - A femoral catheter is a temporary vascular access placed in the femoral vein in the groin. The femoral vein is easy to reach and preserves blood vessels in the upper body for permanent vascular access. However, the site is very prone to infection and limits the patient's mobility. Therefore, it is typically used for critically ill or bedridden patients.

**FEMORAL VEIN** - A continuation of the popliteal vein upward toward the external iliac vein.

**FERRITIN** - Ferritin is an iron storage protein complex that occurs in body tissues and is measured with a blood test. Adequate ferritin stores are necessary to help ensure that EPOGEN can be effectively utilized to stimulate red blood cell production.

**FIBER BUNDLE VOLUME (FBV)** - Fiber bundle volume, also called total cell volume (TCV), is a measure of the volume of fluid that the hollow fibers in a dialyzer can hold. Fiber bundle volume is measured before a dialyzer is used for the first time and again after each reprocessing, because reprocessing a dialyzer can alter the FBV. (*See also: Reprocessing*).

**FIBRIN** - A whitish filamentous protein formed by the action of thrombin or fibrogen. The fibrin is deposited, as fine interlacing filaments is which are entangled red and white blood cells and platelets, the whole forming a coagulum or clot.

**FIBRIN SHEATH** - A fibrin sheath is a collection of blood clotting fibers on the outside of a catheter lumen. The fibers can form a cap that blocks the end of a catheter and reduces blood flow. (*See also: Catheter, Lumen*).

**FIBROSIS** - Fibrosis is the overgrowth of scar tissue. Fibrosis can develop in a fistula as a result of repeated needle punctures for dialysis. The scar tissue builds up, gradually narrowing the lumen of the vessel and reducing the blood flow. (*See also: Arterio Venous Fistula, Lumen*).

**FILTERS** - Filters are devices that remove particles, solutes, and other substances of a given size by passing them through holes of various sizes. Sediment filters are components of dialysis water treatment systems that trap undissolved particles such as sand and mud before they can reach the reverse osmosis membrane and damage it. Depth filters are a type of sediment filter that may contain one or more layers of fibrous material or mesh, each layer finer than the one before, to trap smaller and smaller particles. These filters can remove nearly all-floating particles from the feed water.

**FILTRATION** - Filtration is the process of passing fluid through a filter. In dialysis, filtration forces fluid out of the patient's blood and across the dialyzer membrane by using pressure.

**FIRST USE SYNDROME** - First use syndrome is a group of symptoms that may occur shortly after the beginning of a dialysis treatment with a new dialyzer. Symptoms may include nervousness, chest pain, back pain, palpitations, (skipped or missed heartbeats) or itching. First use syndrome may be caused by exposure to ethylene oxide gas or manufacturing residues remaining in the dialyzer after production. Pre-processing a dialyzer may reduce the incidence of first use syndrome by removing ethylene oxide and manufacturing residues called plasticizers. A coating of blood protein remaining in the dialyzer after dialysis also makes a reprocessed dialyzer more biocompatible—unless the coating is removed by bleach during reprocessing. *(See also: Biocompatible, Cellulose, Ethylene Oxide, and Reprocessing)*.

**FISTULA** - Unnatural opening or passage. In dialysis, the result of anastamosis of an artery to a vein to allow access to the blood stream for hemodialysis. *(See also Arteriovenous Fistula)*.

**FLOCCULANT** - A flocculant is a chemical added to a municipal water supply to make the water clearer. Alum is one substance that may be used a flocculant. (*See also: Alum*).

**FLOW** - Flow is a stream. Blood flow to each organ in the body is determined by the amount and pressure of blood delivered by the heart, and the resistance of the blood meets in the blood vessels. The setting of the blood pump, resistance in the extracorporeal circuit, and capacity of the vascular access determine blood flow in the extracorporeal circuit.

**FLUID DYNAMICS** – A description of how two fluids, blood and dialysate, are pumped through tubing systems. (Within the dialyzer, blood and dialysate are separated from each other by a semipermeable membrane).

**FLUID MOVEMENT** - See osmosis.

**FLUSH** - See priming.

**FOOD AND DRUG ADMINISTRATION (FDA)** - The FDA is a federal office that regulates the release and marketing of medications and medical devices, including dialyzers and devices used for reprocessing.

**FORMALDEHYDE** - Formaldehyde is a poisonous, colorless, foul-smelling gas. In its liquid form (37% gas in water) it is called aqueous formaldehyde or Formalin, and it is an effective germicide used for disinfecting dialysate delivery systems, or for reprocessing dialyzers. The liquid form is volatile, changing readily into vapor that can penetrate and disinfect even small spaces. Formaldehyde is a suspected cancer-causing agent; facilities must follow OSHA safety procedures to prevent injury to patients or staff.

**FORMALIN** - Formalin is a trademark name for a 37% solution of formaldehyde.

**FREE CHLORINE** - Free chlorine is chlorine that is not chemically bound to other substances. (*See also: Chloramines*).

**FRONTAL PLANE** - A plane parallel with the long axis of the body and at right angles to the median sagittal plane. A plane that divides the body into anterior and posterior sections.

**FUNCTIONAL STATUS** - Functional status is an individual's ability to perform usual activities, such as walking, cooking, dressing, toileting, working, attending school, etc.

# DIALYSIS ACRONYMS
# G

# G

**GASTROPARESIS** – Delayed emptying of food from the stomach into the small bowel. Gastroparesis may be a chronic complication of diseases marked by autonomic failure such as diabetes mellitus, chronic renal failure and amyloidosis.

**GERMICIDE** - A germicide is a germ-killing solution. Germicides are used in reprocessing dialyzers. (*See also: Dialyzer, Formalin, Reprocessing, and Solution*).

**GLANDS** - A secretory organ or structure. A cell group or a group of cells that can manufacture a secretion discharged and used in some other part of the body.

**GLOMERULAR FILTRATE** - Glomerular filtrate is a watery fluid left when the blood is filtered by healthy kidneys. It is the protein free plasma from which urine is formed. Low molecular weight substances (small waste particles and water) pass through tiny pores in the glomeruli and into Bowman's space. A healthy adult produces about 180 liters of glomerular filtrate per day. (*See also: Glomerulus*).

**GLOMERULAR FILTRATION** - The process of fluid passing from the blood through the capillary walls of the glomeruli of the kidney to be filtered.

**GLOMERULAR FILTRATION RATE (GFR) -** The GFR is the volume of blood filtered by the glomerulus each minute, in ml/min. A normal GRF is about 120 to 130 ml/min. People with kidney failure have GFR's that are below normal.

**GLOMERULONEPHRITIS -** Glomerulonephritis is an inflammation that damages the glomeruli of the kidneys. Hypertension often accompanies glomerulonephritis. Glomerulonephritis can be slow and progressive or rapid in onset, and sometimes occurs as an immune response to a streptococcal infection. (The incidence of glomerulonephritis has decreased significantly over the past 20 years as a result of earlier treatment of streptococcal infection).

**GLOMERULUS -** The glomerulus is a tangled ball of capillaries that are a part of a kidney nephron. Water and small molecular weight particles are forced through filtration silts in each glomerulus by the pressure of the beating heart. The resulting solution is called glomerular filtrate.

**GRADIENT -** A gradient is a difference. A concentration gradient is a difference in the concentration of solutes of two different fluids, separated by a semipermeable membrane. In dialysis the fluids are blood and dialysate separated by a dialyzer membrane in hemodialysis or by the peritoneum in the peritoneal dialysis.

**GRAFT -** To graft is to join one thing surgically to another. In hemodialysis, a graft is a piece of artificial vessel that can be used to create an access. One end of the graft is connected to the patient's artery, the other to the vein.

**GRAM-NEGATIVE -** Gram-negative bacteria are a class of bacteria that turn pink in a standard laboratory Gram's stain. They have adapted especially to survive in water. These bacteria form an electrically charged bio-film (slime) that allows them to cling to surfaces, such as dialysate containers or hoses. The biofilm protects the bacteria from disinfectants, making them difficult to remove. For example Acromobacter is a Gram-negative bacteria that can contaminate in the dialysis water supply or the dialysate. Acinetobacter, Aeromonas, Alcaligenes, Flavobacterium, Moraxella, Pseudomonas, and Serratia are other types of Gram-Negative bacteria.

**GRAM-POSITIVE BACTERIA -** Gram-positive bacteria turn blue to black in a standard laboratory Gram's stain. Staphylococci are gram-positive bacteria that cause most access infections.

**GUAIAC CARDS -** Guaiac Cards are used to test for hidden (occult) blood in stool. A developing solution is dipped onto a smear of stool on a Guaiac card. If the stain turns blue, blood is present. Guaiac cards may be used with patients with low hematocrit or hemoglobin levels to determine if gastrointestinal bleeding is occurring. (*See also: Anemia*).

# DIALYSIS ACRONYMS
# H

# H

**HARD WATER** - The total concentration of calcium and magnesium in water.

**HEADERS** - A plastic cap covering the ends of the hollow fibers enclosed in the plastic casing (dialyzer).

**HEALTH CARE FINANCING ADMINISTRATION (HCFA)** - HCFA is a federal agency that oversees Medicare and other health related agencies. Dialyzer reprocessing and the related health standards and conditions of reprocessing are also regulated by HCFA.

**HEAT DISINFECTION** - An alternative to chemical disinfectants used to reprocess certain types of dialyzer and to disinfect dialysis equipment (that is equipped with this feature). Heat disinfection prevents patient and staff exposure to chemicals. Cellulose-based dialyzer membranes degrade during heat disinfection, and therefore cannot be disinfected using heat.

**HEMASTIX** - A reagent strip that reacts to the presence of blood. When the blood leak detector indicates the presence of blood in the used dialysate and the blood is not visible, a Hemastix should be used to determine the presence and the extent of the leak. (*See also: Blood Leak Detector, Dialysate*).

**HEMATOCRIT** - A measure of red blood cells in the blood, stated as a percentage of red blood cells per total blood volume. Routinely checking hematocrit levels allows clinicians to assess anemia, follow the patient's response to EPOGEN, and alert the staff to any chronic loss of blood. NKF-DOQI guidelines recommend a target hematocrit level for dialysis patients of 33% to 36%. (*See also: Anemia, EPOGEN, and Hemoglobin*).

**HEMATOMA** - A painful, hard, discolored (black-and-blue) collection of blood under the skin, caused by blood escaping from a vessel into surrounding tissue. Hematomas can form during or after placement of dialysis needles and when needles are removed.

**HEMOCONCENTRATION** - The dehydration of the blood, which can occur in the extracorporeal circuit if ultrafiltration continues after the blood pump is turned off, or if recirculation within the access is occurring. Hemoconcentration can lead to blood clotting.

**HEMODIALYSIS** - A process that cleans the blood of waste products by passing the blood through an artificial kidney, or dialyzer. Blood and dialysate are passed through the membrane, and into the dialysate according to the principles of diffusion and osmosis. Hemodialysis is the most commonly chosen treatment modality for patients with end-stage renal disease.

**HEMODIALYSIS ADEQUACY** - A measure of the dose of dialysis a patient receives to be sure enough dialysis is given to allow the patient to feel well and have a good quality of life. The first clinical practice guidelines, developed by the Renal Physicians Association (RPA).

**HEMODIALYSIS DELIVERY SYSTEM** - A machine that consists of a blood pump, dialysis solution, dialysate, delivery system, and appropriate safety monitors. The blood pump moves blood from the patient's access side through the dialyzer and back to the patient. The machine prepares dialysate by mixing specially treated water with the dialysate concentrate. The delivery system also controls and monitors dialysate conductivity, temperature, flow rate, and pressure. (*See also: Extracorporeal Circuit*).

**HEMODIALYZER** - See dialyzer.

**HEMOGLOBIN** - Hemoglobin is the oxygen-carrying pigment of red blood cells. Measuring hemoglobin levels is a means of diagnosing anemia. Routinely checking hemoglobin levels allows clinicians to follow the patient's response to EPOGEN and alerts the staff to any chronic blood loss. NKF-DOQI guidelines recommend a target hemoglobin range of between 11 and 12 g/dl. The EPOGEN package insert recommends a target hemoglobin range of 10 to 12 g/dl. (*See also: Anemia, EPOGEN*).

**HEMOLYSIS** - The destruction of red blood cells by bursting, a life-threatening condition that requires immediate attention from a physician. Hemolysis may be caused by hyponatremia (low blood sodium); overheated dialysate; too diluted (hypotonic) dialysate; chloramines, copper, or nitrates in the dialysate water; formaldehyde or bleach in the dialysate; low-conductivity (too much water and not enough concentrate); too high prepump arterial pressure; incompatible blood transfusions; occlusion or kinking of blood tubing; some medications; and certain diseases.

**HEMOLYTIC ANEMIA** - Anemia resulting from hemolysis of red blood cells acquired from the effects of toxic agents.

**HEMOTHORAX** - A collection of blood in the chest that prevents the lungs from fully expanding, causing difficulty breathing. Hemothorax can occur if a blood vessel is accidentally punctured during placement of a dialysis catheter.

**HEPARIN** - An anticoagulant or an anticlotting medication, given during dialysis to allow blood to flow freely through the extracorporeal circuit.

**HEPARIN INFUSION LINE** - The heparin line is a very small in diameter tube that extends out of the blood tubing that allows the administration of heparin during dialysis. The heparin infusion line is normally located on the arterial blood-tubing segment just before the dialyzer.

**HEPARIN PUMP** - A heparin fusion pump consists of a syringe holder, a piston, and an electric motor, and is used to continuously to deliver precise amounts of heparin during dialysis. The heparin pump is connected to the heparin infusion line, which is part of the extracorporeal blood tubing. Most dialysis machines produced today include a heparin delivery system, although stand-alone heparin pumps are still in use in some settings.

**HEPATITIS** - Hepatitis is an inflammation of the liver caused by a virus that can be found in several forms, including hepatitis viruses A, B (HBV) or C (HCV). Because hepatitis B and C are spread through contact with infected blood or other body fluid, they are a concern for hemodialysis patients and staff. Hepatitis virus infections can cause long-term and permanent liver damage or death. Vaccination against the hepatitis B virus should be offered to all dialysis staff members and patients. Standard precautions should be followed to prevent the spread of hepatitis, as well as other infections.

**HEPATORENAL SYNDROME** - Condition in which the patient exhibits both kidney and liver failure.

**HIGH-EFFICIENCY DIALYSIS** - High efficiency dialysis uses dialyzers that are capable of removing more small solutes (i.e., urea) than conventional membranes. Blood flow rates ranging from 300 to 500 ml/min are usually used, as well as having UF control when dialysis is done with a dialyzer's KUF above 8. (*See also: Coefficient of Ultrafiltration*).

**HIGH-EFFICIENCY DIALYZER** – Dialyzers with medium to large surface areas (1.3 – 2.2 square meters), medium KUFs (8 – 12 ml/mmHg/hr) and low molecular weight cutoffs (3,000 Daltons). These dialyzers can be made of cellulose or synthetic material and must be used with ultrafiltration control machines. (*See also: High-efficiency dialysis*).

**HIGH-FLUX DIALYSIS** - High-flux dialysis uses a membrane permeable to a broad range of molecular weight solutes, including higher molecular weight solutes. Kuf's for high-flux dialysis are higher than 8, making ultrafiltration control mandatory. High-flux dialyzers have the ability to remove larger amounts of fluid as well as large substances such as beta-2-microglobulin or $B_2M$.

**HIGH-FLUX DIALYZER** – Dialyzers with medium too large surface areas (up to 2.0 square meters), high KUFs (12 – 60+ ml/mmHg/hr) and high molecular weight cutoffs (15,000 Daltons). These dialyzers are made of synthetic material and tend to be more biocompatible. These dialyzers must, also, be used with ultrafiltration control machines. (*See also: High-flux dialysis*).

**HIGH-OUTPUT CARDIAC FAILURE** – Condition that occurs when the patient's heart grows larger, but still cannot work hard enough to pump out the extra blood sent to the heart by placement of an AV fistula or graft. (*See also: Cardiac Output*).

**HISTOLOGY** - The study of microscopic structure of tissue.

**HOLOW FIBER** – Dialyzer membrane material (cellulose or synthetic) formed into thin tubes enclosed in a plastic case that holds the dialyzer together and provides pathways for blood and dialysate to flow in and out of the dialyzer.

**HOLLOW FIBER DIALYZER** - The hollow fiber dialyzer contains thousands of tiny hollow fibers (semipermeable membranes), held in place at each end by clay-like potting material. The hollow fiber and potting material are encased in a hard plastic cylinder. During dialysis the blood flows through the hollow tubes, and dialysate is circulated around them. The hollow fiber dialyzer allows for well-controlled and predictable diffusion and ultrafiltration, and is currently the only type of dialyzer available in the U.S. (*See also: Dialyzer, Diffusion, and Ultrafiltration*).

**HOMEOSTASIS** - The relatively constant balance naturally maintained in the internal environment of the body. Healthy kidneys help maintain fluid balance, acid/base balance, hormonal balance, and electrolyte balance, all-important component of homeostasis.

**HORMONES** - Chemical substances produced on one organ or gland of the body that act on a different organ. Healthy kidneys produce a hormone (erythropoietin) that causes red blood cells to be manufactured by the bone marrow, and other hormones that maintain blood pressure and regulate calcium metabolism.

**HUMAN IMMUNODEFICIENCY VIRUS (HIV)** - A virus that disables the body's immune system by destroying white blood cells that fight disease (T-lymphocytes). HIV is transmitted through blood, semen, vaginal secretions, peritoneal fluids, and breast milk, Over time, people infected with HIV can develop immunodeficiency syndrome (AIDS). Damage to the immune system caused by AIDS leaves the body vulnerable to infections and cancers the usually do not occur in people with healthy immune systems. While new treatments are available, prevention is the best approach. Follow standard precautions to prevent the spread of HIV in the dialysis unit. (*See also: Infection Control, Opportunistic Illness, and Standard Precautions*).

**HYDRAULIC PRESSURE** - Water pressure created naturally (such as from gravity) or artificially (such as from a pump). Hydraulic pressure is one factor that affects the amount of water that will be removed from the patient during dialysis.

**HYDROSTATIC PRESSURE** - Pressure produced by the height of a column of fluid.

**HYPER** - The prefix hyper means beyond, above, more, or too much. For example, hyperactivity is an above normal activity level.

**HYPERCALCEMIA** – Means too much calcium (an electrolyte) in the blood. Patient symptoms of hypercalcemia can include muscle weakness, fatigue, constipation, loss of appetite, abdominal cramps, nausea, vomiting, and coma. (*See also: Electrolyte*).

**HYPERKALEMIA** - Means too much potassium (an electrolyte) in the blood. Hyperkalemia causes symptoms of muscle weakness, and can lead to cardiac arrhythmias, cardiac arrest, or death. Hyperkalemia can occur if the dialysis patient eats too man high potassium foods; if there is tissue breakdown due to surgery, bleeding, hemolysis, or fever; or if dialysate with too much potassium is used. These conditions cause potassium to be released from cells into the bloodstream. (*See also: Electrolyte*).

**HYPERMAGNESEMIA** - Means too much magnesium (an electrolyte) in the blood.

Magnesium is needed for muscle and nerve functioning. Symptoms of hypermagnesmia include impaired nerve transmission, hypotension, respiratory depression, and sleepiness. Severe hypermagnesmia can cause cardiac arrest. (*See also: Electrolyte*).

**HYPERNATREMIA** - Means too much sodium (an electrolyte) in the blood. Excess sodium in the blood causes water to move out of the cells—including red blood cells – and into the extracellular space. Hypernatremia can cause headaches, hypertension, and crenation, a shrinkage of red blood cells that can be fatal. (*See also: Electrolyte*).

**HYPERPARATHYROID BONE DISEASE** – A bone disease or condition resulting from over activity of the parathyroid glands causing excessive levels of parathyroid hormone (PTH) in the body with resulting disturbances in calcium and phosphorus metabolism. It is characterized by decalcification of the bone, elevated levels of blood calcium, lowering levels of blood phosphorus, and kidney stones.

**HYPERPHOSPHATEMIA** - Means too much phosphorus in the blood. Phosphorous is a component of bones, and is also key in energy transfer between cells. When combined with hypercalcemia, hyperphosphatemia can cause crystal deposits in soft tissues, fractures and bone pain. Hyperphosphatemia is usually found in patients who are eating more than the prescribed amount of protein and or dairy products, not taking enough phosphate binders, or not timing the ingestion of phosphate binders to coincide with their meals.

**HYPERPLASIA** – Is the overgrowth of cells. Clotting that occurs in the middle of a vascular access graft is often caused by clumps of platelets developing on areas of hyperplasia.

**HYPERSENSITIVITY** - An excessive or abnormal sensitivity or allergy. Hypersensitivity reactions occur most often with cuprophane dialyzer, and can even lead to anaphylaxis in some patients. (*See also: Anaphylactic Reaction*).

**HYPERTENSION** - Means high blood pressure. In the adult, a condition in which the B/P is higher than 140/90 on three separate readings recorded several weeks apart. Hypertension can be a cause or a result of kidney failure; it is the second most common cause of kidney disease in the U.S. Hypertension can damage the kidneys, heart, blood vessels, and other organs.

**HYPO** - The prefix "hypo" means below, beneath or too little. For example, hypocalcemia means there is too little calcium in the blood. A hypodermic needle is a needle that is inserted below the skin.

**HYPOCALCEMIA** - Means not enough calcium (an electrolyte) in the blood). Hypocalcemia can cause tetany—spasms and twitching of the muscles or seizures. Low blood calcium can occur in kidney disease due to the loss of calcitrol production by the failing kidneys. Calcitrol allows the body to absorb calcium from the diet. (*See also: Electrolyte*).

**HYPOKALEMIA** - Means not enough potassium (an electrolyte) in the blood. This condition is unusual in dialysis patients, but can occur when there is not enough potassium in the diet or dialysate. Hypokalemia can also be caused by a loss of potassium, due to vomiting, diarrhea, use of potassium exchange resins, and use of diuretics that can increase the loss of potassium in the urine. (*See also: Electrolyte*).

**HYPONATREMIA** - Means not enough sodium (an electrolyte) in the blood. Without enough sodium, water moves out of the extracellular space and into cells, which can cause hypotension, muscle cramps, and hemolysis—destruction of red blood cells. (*See also: Electrolyte*).

**HYPOPHOSPHATEMIA** - Means not enough phosphorous in the blood. This condition is rare in dialysis patients, because phosphorous is found in most foods. Predisponding factors include poor nutritional intake and excessive intake of phosphate binders. Low levels of phosphorous can indicate malnutrition. Serious consequences of hypophosphatemia include cardiac arrhythmias or muscle weakness.

**HYPOTENSION** - Blood pressure that is abnormally low. A decrease of the B/P below normal, less than 100/60. In dialysis patients, hypotension occurs most commonly when too much fluid is removed during dialysis, or when patients are overmedicated with antihypertensive drugs. Symptoms of hypotension include feeling of warmth, restlessness, dizziness, nausea, or visual disturbance. The trendelenberg—raising the feet higher than the heart—and volume replacement (i.e., normal saline) help relieve hypotension.

**HYPOTONIC DIALYSATE** - Hypotonic dialysate is dialysate that is diluted with too much water, which can lead to hemolysis. (*See also: Hemolysis*).

# **DIALYSIS ACRONYMS**
# I

# I

**IMMUNOSUPPRESSIVE DRUGS** - Drugs used to reduce the severity of immune reactions to such substances as protein.

**IN-CENTER HEMODIALYSIS** - Treatments are performed in a hospital or freestanding dialysis clinic. In-center dialysis is usually assisted by dialysis staff members, although patients may be able to take their own vital signs, place their own needles, and monitor their own treatments.

**INFECTION** - A condition produced by invasion of the body with a disease-producing organism (i.e., bacteria).

**INFECTION CONTROL** - A series of steps taken to prevent the spread of infection. Using aseptic technique for invasive procedures, disinfecting equipment after use, washing hands, and wearing protective equipment are all part of infection control. (*See also: Standard Precautions*).

**INFILTRATION** - An abnormal leakage of a substance into bodily tissues. In dialysis patients, infiltration of blood into the tissues surrounding the vascular access can occur if the needle punctures the back of the vessel wall. To prevent infiltration, needle insertion must be performed carefully.

**INFLAMMATION** - Tissue swelling in reaction to injury, infection, or surgery.

**INORGANIC-** Chemical compounds that do not contain carbon. Non-living bacteria.

**INSTILL** - To place into or to cause to enter. Heparin is instilled into each lumen of a catheter to prevent clotting in the catheter between dialysis treatments. PD fluid is instilled into the peritoneum for peritoneal dialysis.

**INTEGRITY** – Unimpaired, undiminished state (Pure state).

**INTERDIALYTIC** - Means between dialysis treatments. Patients must restrict their fluid intake to prevent interdialytic fluid gain that complicates fluid removal during a single hemodialysis treatment.

**INTERMITTENT** - Means "periodically" or not "continuously". Heparin can be given intermittently throughout dialysis. (*See also: Heparin*).

**INTERNAL JUGULAR CATHETER (IJ)** - Temporary or permanent dialysis catheters placed in the internal jugular vein in the neck. This location is less likely to cause central venous stenosis than placement in the subclavian vein. (*See also: Central Venous Stenosis*).

**INTERNAL JUGULAR VEIN** - Any of the two bilateral veins located in the neck that return blood from the head to the heart. In dialysis these veins are used for placement of temporary or permanent dialysis catheters.

**INTERSTITIAL FLUID** - Fluid that surrounds the cells, in tissue spaces. Tissue fluid.

**INTERSTITIAL SPACE** - The space between the cells of an organ or tissue.

**INTIMA** - The smooth lining of the inner surfaces of arteries and veins. The intima is covered with a thin, fragile layer of cells that allows blood to flow through the vessel easily.

**INTRACELLULAR** - Means within the cells. Sodium causes fluid to move across cell membranes between the intracellular and extracellular spaces. (*See also: Extracellular*).

**INTRACELLULAR FLUID** – Fluid within the cell, approximately 2/3 of body water.

**INTRADERMAL** - Means within the skin. Local anesthetics may be injected intradermally.

**INTRAMUSCULAR** - Means within the muscle.

**INTRAVASCULAR** - Means with in blood vessels.

**INTRAVENOUS** - Intravenous means within the vein. Many medications, including EPOGEN, are injected intravenously.

**INVITRO** - Invitro is a Latin phrase that means outside the human body and in an artificial environment. Dialyzer clearance is measured invitro by the manufacturer; using non-blood fluids (i.e., saline), so actual dialyzer clearance may vary from the manufactures' specifications.

**INVIVO** - Invivo is a Latin phrase that means within the plant or animal. Tests performed on a dialyzer while a patient is being treated are considered invivo.

**ION** – Electrically charged particles; electrolytes. Ions are formed when electrons in the outer shell are either gained or lost. Ions carry a positive charge (cation) or a negative charge (anion).

**ION EXCHANGE** - A process that occurs inside a deionizer for water treatment. Unwanted ions are traded for hydrogen and hydroxyl ions to create pure water. (*See also: Deionizer*).

**IRON DEFICIENCY** - A lack of sufficiently available iron in the body to make red blood cells. Without iron, which is needed to synthesize hemoglobin, bone marrow cannot make red blood cells, even if erythropoietin levels are sufficient. Low levels of iron can cause a form of anemia. (*See also: Anemia*).

**ISCHEMIA** - The lack of sufficient oxygen to the tissues, due to reduced blood flow. The affected tissues may have pain. For example, ischemia of the heart can cause angina pain; ischemia of the hand may include symptoms of hand pain during exercise, a cold, clammy feeling and in extreme cases, painful, non-healing skin ulcers. Limb ischemia can be caused by placement or complications of some vascular accesses, and, in severe cases, can lead to loss of a limb.

**ISOLATED ULTRAFILTRATION (IU)** - An extracorporeal treatment that removes water, but not solutes, by using the extracorporeal circuit and dialyzer without dialysate. IU is also called dry ultrafiltration, sequential ultrafiltration, or pure ultrafiltration. Isolated ultrafiltration can be performed before, after, or independently of dialysis. The principle advantage of IU is that fluid removal is better tolerated that with conventional hemodialysis.

**ISOTONIC** - Having the same concentration or the same osmotic pressure.

# DIALYSIS ACRONYMS
# K

# K

**KIDNEY** - Paired organs, purple brown in color, situated at the back of the abdominal cavity, one on each side of the spinal column. Their function is to excrete the urine and to help regulate the water, electrolyte, and acid based content of the blood.

**KIDNEY TRANSPLANT** - A replacement of a diseased kidney with a healthy kidney from a donor. Only one healthy kidney is needed to live. It is possible to receive a donor kidney from a relative, spouse or friend, or a cadaver (deceased). Blood type and other tissue factors are used to "match" a recipient after a medical work-up has been done.

**Kt/V** – Formula used to determine the actual delivered dose of dialysis. (*See also: Urea Kinetic Modeling, Natural Logarithm*).

**KUF** – Means the manufacturer's specified ultrafiltration coefficient. The KUF is the amount of fluid removed by the dialyzer in one hour at a given pressure; stated as ml/mmHg/hr. (*See also: Coefficient of Ultrafiltration*).

# DIALYSIS ACRONYMS
# L

# L

**LABEL (on a REUSE DIALYZER)** - The label consists of the name of the patient, the number of times the dialyzer has been reprocessed, the date and time of the last reprocess, the original residual, the total cell or fiber bundle volume, the signature of the person who performed the reprocessing, and the initials of the tech that puts the patient on dialysis.

**LAMINAR FLOW** - Streamlined flow of a viscous fluid near a solid boundary.

**LEACH** - Occurs when a fluid passes through a substance and dissolves away part of that substance. In water treatment, copper lead, or galvanized steel pipes should not be used after the blending valve because water can leach copper from the copper pipes, or zinc from the galvanized pipes.

**LEAK TESTING** - See Pressure Testing.

**LEUKOCYTE** - White blood corpuscle or blood cells. There are two types: granulocytes, and agranulocytes.

**LIDOCAINE** - A local anesthetic drug. Trade name is Xylocaine.

**LOADING DOSE** - A dose of medication that creates a certain level in the body. A loading dose of heparin may be given after both needles are in place, but before the treatment begins, to allow that heparin to circulate throughout the patient's body.

**LOCAL INFECTION** - An infection only in one specific area—such as in a blood vessel or graft and the surrounding tissues.

**LOOP OF HENLE** – Part of the nephron; the descending and ascending loops of the renal tubule, between the proximal convoluted tubule and the distal convoluted tubule.

**LUMEN** - The lumen is the inside diameter of a tube (i.e., catheter or needle) or a tubular organ (i.e., an artery or vein). In stenosis, the lumen of the vascular access becomes narrower, limiting the blood flow.

**LYSE** - To lyse is to dissolve. One option for treating a blood clot in a vascular access is to use a medication that will lyse the clot.

# DIALYSIS ACRONYMS
# M

# M

**MAGNESIUM** - A metallic mineral. It is found in the body as an electrolyte in the intracellular fluid; a small trace of magnesium in body fluids is essential to the function of the nervous system. (*See also: Dialysate*).

**MASTER FILE OR MASTER RECORD** - Summary of all reprocessing procedures, specifications, policies and procedures, training materials, manuals, and methods for reprocessing.

**MATERIAL SAFETY DATA SHEET (MSDS)** - Prepared and supplied by the manufacturer of the chemical, it contains information on that chemical and corrective action to take in the event of a spill or exposure.

**MATTER** - Anything that occupies a space, may be gaseous or solid.

**MEDICARE ESRD PROGRAM** - Was established by the U.S. congress in 1972. The program extended Medicare benefits to the patients with renal disease that were entitled to Social Security Benefits. The ESRD program pays for 80% of the allowable cost of dialysis treatment for eligible patients.

**MEMBRANE FILTERS** - Membrane filters are water treatment cartridges containing thin membranes with pores of a specified size. Membrane filters remove small particles and some solutes.

**METABOLIC ACIDOSIS** - A condition in which the acid/base balance of a body fluid has shifted toward acidic because there is a build-up of acid in the body. Dialysis patients commonly develop metabolic acidosis, because their kidneys no longer appropriately reabsorb bicarbonate—a blood buffer that stabilizes blood pH. For this reason, bicarbonate is usually used as a buffer for dialysate. (*See also: Bicarbonate, Buffer*).

**METABOLISM** - The sum of chemical processes that involve breaking down some substances and creating other substances.

**METASTATIC CALCIFICATION** - See Extraskeletal Calcification.

**MICROALBUMINURIA** - The presence of tiny amounts of albumin in the urine. This condition, measured by a simple urine test, can be an early indicator of chronic renal failure, because albumin is too large a molecule to pass through healthy glomeruli. A class of blood pressure medications called ACE inhibitors, such as catopril, has been shown to slow progression of kidney failure is diabetic patients with microalbuminuria. (*See also: Albumin*).

**MICRONS** - The unit of measure for filter pores. Filters with high micron sizes trap large particles and allow smaller particles to flow through. A submicron filter may be required to capture very small particles. (*See also: Filters*).

**MICROORGANISMS** - Living things too small to be seen without a microscope. Algae, fungi, bacteria, and viruses are types of microorganisms. Some microorganisms can cause illness if they enter the body. Bacteria are important sources of microorganism contamination for dialysis patients. (*See also: Bacteria*).

**MIDDLE MOLECULES** - Molecules with a molecular weight in the range of 300 to 2,000 that diffuse poorly across conventional membranes. Molecules in this range are suspected of being a cause of uremic neuropathogenicity.

**MODALITY** - A type of treatment such as hemodialysis, peritoneal dialysis, or transplantation.

**MOLECULAR WEIGHT** - A measure of the size of a molecule. Weight of a molecule attained by totaling the atomic weight of its constituent atoms. Molecular weight is measured in Daltons. Large molecules (like beta-2-microglobulin) have high molecular weights.

**MOLECULAR WEIGHT CUTOFF -** The solute range that can pass through a particular semipermeable membrane.

**MOLECULE** - The smallest complete unit of a substance that retains that substance's identity.

**MORBIDITY -** Illness. Morbidity sometimes measured as days of hospitalization, is used as one measure of patient outcomes.

**MORTALITY -** Death. Mortality is used as one measure of patient outcomes.

**MYALGIA -** Muscle pain.

**MYOCARDIAL INFRACTION -** The blockage of a heart artery, which can lead to death in part of the heart muscle. The patient may feel severe or crushing chest pain—a "heart attack". Myocardial infraction is commonly abbreviates as MI. *(See also: Arrhythmia)*.

# DIALYSIS ACRONYMS
# N

# N

**NASOGASTRIC (NG) TUBE** - A tube that is inserted through the nose into the stomach. Patients who are extremely malnourished may need to be fed through the NG tube.

**NEGATIVE PRESSURE** - Pressure that is less than 0 mmHg, created by suction, or a vacuum. In dialysis, negative pressure is created by a pump, which pulls fluid from the blood compartment. Negative pressure plus positive pressure equals transmembrane pressure. (*See also: Positive Pressure, Transmembrane Pressure, and Ultrafiltration*).

**NEOINTIMAL HYPERPLASIA** - Occurs when smooth muscle cells at the venous anastomosis form extra layers of cells that fill up the graft lumen, reducing blood flow. (*See also: Anastomosis, Lumen*).

**NEPHROLOGIST** - A doctor who specializes in kidney disease.

**NEPHROLOGY** - The study of the kidneys. As a medical specialty, nephrology deals with information, care, and knowledge of kidneys. A nephrologist is a doctor of internal medicine who specializes in nephrology. A pediatrician nephrologist is a physician who specializes in the care of children and adolescents with kidney disease. A nephrology nurse has a special training in the care of people with renal failure. A nephrology technician has training in the care of people with renal failure and the technology that supports their care.

**NEPHRONS** - Tiny blood purification filters contained in the kidneys. Nephrons filter all of the waste products from the body, and maintain electrolyte and fluid balance. Each kidney contains approximately one million microscopic nephrons. Each nephron has its own tiny blood vessels (capillaries) that supply it with blood to be cleaned. Each nephron is made up of a glomerulus and tubules. (*See also: Glomerulus*).

**NEUROPATHY -** See Peripheral Neuropathy.

**NKF-DOQI (NATIONAL KIDNEY FOUNDATION – DIALYSIS OUTCOMES QUALITY INITIATIVE) CLINICAL PRACTICE GUIDELINES -** See Clinical Practice Guidelines.

**NON-POTABLE** - Not suitable for consumption (drinking).

**NORMAL SALINE -** A sterile salt-water solution containing 0.9% sodium chloride, equal to the concentration of sodium chloride found in the blood. In hemodialysis, normal saline is needed to prime and prepare the extracorporeal circuit, and is used for fluid replacement during the treatment.

**NO TRANSFER LEVEL** – Limits set by AAMI for trace metals in water used for dialysis treatment. A level low enough so that none of the substances will transfer from dialysate into the patient's blood. (i.e., lead, mercury, arsenic, silver).

**NOSOCOMIAL** - Means hospital acquired. The term is usually applied to infections or illnesses patients acquire during the course of their medical treatment while in the hospital or nursing home environment.

# DIALYSIS ACRONYMS
# O

# O

**OLIGURIA** – Urinary output of less than 400 cc/day; usually results in renal failure if not reversed. Seen after profuse perspiration, bleeding, diarrhea, and renal failure due to any disease. Also in retention disease of the central nervous system, shock, drug poisoning, deep coma, or hypertrophy of the prostate.

**OPPORTUNISTIC ILLNESSES** - Occurs when a patient's immune system is impaired, or weakened. Patients with AIDS, for example, are vulnerable to opportunistic infections because their immune systems have been compromised.

**ORGAN** - A part of the body having a special function. Many organs are in pairs. In such pairs, one organ may be extirpated and the remaining one can perform all necessary functions peculiar to it. One-third to two fifths of some organs may be removed without loss of function necessary to support life.

**ORGANIC** - Chemical substances that contain carbon.

**ORGAN SYSTEM** – A group of organs related to each other and performing a certain functions together (i.e., digestive system).

**ORTHOSTATIC HYPOTENSION** - A drop in blood pressure of 15 mmHg or more when a person rises from a sitting to standing position.

**OSHA (OCCUPATIONAL SAFETY HEALTH ASSOCIATION)** - A federal agency that oversees safety and health regulations for employees in the work place. Occupational exposure to blood borne pathogens (HBV, HIV). Occupational exposure to formaldehyde and other chemicals. Hazards communications (MSDS).

**OSMOSIS** - The movement of fluid across a semipermeable membrane from an area of lower solute concentration (like blood) to and area of high solute concentration (like dialysate) until the solute concentrations on both sides of the membrane are equal. Natural osmosis is too slow to produce enough fluid removal for hemodialysis, so fluid movement is aided with a hydraulic pressure gradient.

**OSMOTIC GRADIENT** - A difference in concentration of solutes on each side of a semipermeable membrane.

**OSMOTIC PRESSURE** - Is an osmotic gradient created by using dialysate containing substances, such as glucose, that cause fluid to move out of the blood and into the dialysate. (*See also: Dialysate, Osmosis*).

**OSTEOSCLEROSIS** – An abnormal increase in thickening and density of the bone.

**OSTETITIS FIBROSA CYSTICA** – See hyperparathyroid bone disease.

**OXIDANTS** – Chemicals used for disinfection in the reprocessing of dialyzers, such as bleach, renalin, hydrogen peroxide and amuchina; they combine with oxygen to breakdown cell walls killing bacteria.

**OXIDIZERS** - Chemicals combined with oxygen to break down cell walls. (*See also: Oxidants*).

# DIALYSIS ACRONYMS
# P

# P

**PALPATE** - To exam by touch; to feel.

**PALPITATIONS** - Are occasional, strong heartbeats that can be a symptom of cardiac arrhythmia.

**PARATHYROID HORMONE (PTH)** - A hormone produced by four parathyroid glands located in the neck. PTH is released into the bloodstream in the large amounts when the calcium levels are low—a common problem in patients with renal failure—or when levels of phosphorous in the bloodstream are high. Too much PTH can cause hyperparathyroid bone disease. The synthetic form of calcitriol is given to most dialysis patients to help them avoid bone disease. (*See also: Calcium*).

**PATENCY** - The state of openness or the lack of obstruction of a blood vessel or catheter. Before beginning dialysis, patency of the patient's internal access should be checked by listening for the bruit, or feeling for the thrill. (*See also: Access, Bruit, Thrill*).

**PATHOGEN** - An agent (such as bacteria) that causes disease in humans. (*See also: Bacteria*).

**PATHOLOGY -** The study of the nature of the cause of disease, which involves changes in structure and function.

**PATIENT OUTCOMES -** Are the results of care. Morbidity and mortality are traditionally measured outcomes, but other outcomes such as "functional status"—the ability to do usual activities (activities of daily living, or ADLs)—are gaining in importance. Successful rehabilitation is also a patient outcome.

**PERICARDIAL EFFUSION -** A build-up of fluid in the pericardium, or sac surrounding the heart. In severe cases, pericardial infusion can lead to cardiac tamponade, a potentially life threatening condition in which fluid pressure makes it difficult or impossible for the heart to beat.

**PERICARDITIS -** An inflammation of the pericardium, the membrane, or sac that surrounds the heart. Pericarditis causes low-grade fever, hypotension, and persistent pain in the center of the chest that may be relieved by sitting up and taking deep breaths. Patients who are uremic or inadequately dialyzed may be prone to pericarditis.

**PERICIARDIUM -** The double membranous fibroserous sac enclosing the heart and the origins of the great blood vessels. It is composed of an inner serous layer and outer fibrous layer.

**PERIPHERAL** - Means away from the center of the body.

**PERIPHERAL NEUROPATHY** - Neuropathy is nerve damage. Peripheral neuropathy includes symptoms of numbness, tingling, burning, pain and weakness in the hands and feet. In dialysis patients, neuropathy may be caused by one or more toxins retained in uremia and inadequately removed by hemodialysis. Neuropathy may also be a result of vascular access problems, which may lead to waste build-up due to inadequate dialysis. Many cases of peripheral neuropathy can be prevented or treated with adequate dialysis and adherence to diet.

**PERIPHERAL VASCULAR RESISTANCE** - Is a measure of the ability of blood to flow through the blood vessels. A decrease in peripheral resistance (relaxation of blood vessels) will reduce blood pressure if the heart cannot compensate. An increase in peripheral vascular resistance (narrowing of blood vessels) will increase the blood pressure.

**PERITONEAL DIALYSIS (PD)** - Is a type of dialysis that uses the peritoneum (a blood vessel rich sac surrounding the abdominal organs) as a semipermeable membrane. A catheter is surgically inserted into the abdominal cavity to allow sterile dialysate to fill the abdomen, dwell, and drain out. During the dwell time, wastes and excess fluid move from the blood across the peritoneum and into the dialysate by diffusion and osmosis. The peritoneal membrane in the abdomen functions in the same way as the semipermeable membrane in the dialyzer. (*See also: Dwell time*).

**PERITONEUM** - Is a smooth, thin layer of tissue rich in blood vessels, which covers the outside of all the abdominal organs and the inside of the abdominal walls. The peritoneum forms a closed system, somewhat like a sac, and can be used as a semipermeable membrane and the container for dialysate, in the peritoneal dialysis. (*See also: Peritoneal Dialysis*).

**PERITONITIS** - Is a painful infection of the peritoneum. In people on peritoneal dialysis peritonitis is a complication that can occurs when sterile technique is not properly followed during an exchange. (*See also: Peritoneal Dialysis, Sterile*).

**PERMEABILITY** - The quality of being permeable; capable of allowing the passage of fluids or substances in a solution. The property or state of allowing the passage of certain substances.

**PERMEABLE** - Means allowing substances to pass through. Cell membranes in the human body are freely permeable to water, letting fluid pass in and out. Hemodialyzer membranes have varying degrees of permeability, depending on the type of material used and the manufacturing technique; they are semipermeable.

**pH** - Is an expression of the hydrogen ion (acid) concentration of a solution. A solution with a pH above 7 is alkaline, or base; a solution with a pH below 7 is an acid. A solution with a pH of 7.0 is neutral. Normal body pH ranges between 7.35 and 7.45, slightly alkaline. It is important for the pH of dialysate to be within the acceptable range. Bicarbonate-buffered dialysate should have a pH of 7.2 to prevent bacterial growth and the formation of precipitation that could damage equipment. AAMI recommends that water with a pH between 6.0 and 8.0 be used to mix dialysate. (*See also: AAMI, Acid, Base, Bicarbonate*).

**PHOSPHATE BINDERS** - Medications that bind with phosphorous in food so the phosphorous is not absorbed into the bloodstream, but calcium can be absorbed. Phosphorous is then eliminated in the stool. Patients should take more binders with larger meals, fewer binders with small meals or snacks.

**PHOSPHOROUS** - A non-metallic element present in dairy products, meat, poultry, fish, nuts, peanuts, chocolate, and colas. Phosphorous is difficult to avoid in the diet, and damaged kidneys have a difficult time removing it from the blood. Too much phosphorous in the blood can cause secondary hyperparathyroidism and bone disease. Phosphorous levels are checked monthly before dialysis, and most people with renal failure take phosphate binders to control phosphorous. (*See also: Secondary Hyperparathyroidism*).

**PHYSIOLOGY** - The science of the function of the living organisms and its components and of the chemical and physical processes involved.

**PLASTICIZER** - Is a chemical that makes plastic flexible. Priming the dialyzer and blood tubing before use will help clear them of residual plasticizers. (*See also: Priming*).

**PLASMA** - The liquid part of the lymph and of the blood.

**PLATELETS** - Blood cells that promote clotting by clumping together when "activated" by signals sent by injured cells.

**PNEUMOTHORAX** - Is air in the chest cavity that prevents the lungs from expanding. Pneumothorax can occur during central venous catheter placement if the catheter punctures a blood vessel and passes into the space between the lungs and the chest wall.

**POLYMER** - A polymer is a long string of small molecules that's similar to plastic used to make dialyzer semipermeable membranes. (i.e., cellulose polymer, synthetic polymer).

**POLYCYSTIC KIDNEY DISEASE (PKD)** - An inherited disease that causes large, fluid-filled cysts to develop in the kidneys. The cysts can even become so large and numerous that they crowd out normal kidney tissue, which can cause kidney failure.

**PORES** - Pores are holes. In a semipermeable dialyzer membrane, membrane filter, or reverse osmosis unit, the size of the pores is designed to allow solutes of a certain size range to pass through, while trapping solutes that are too large to fit through.

**POSITIONAL** - Means affected by the patient's body position. When hemodialysis catheters are positional, blood flow can be interrupted or decreased by the patient's movement. If the patient coughs or changes position, the blood flow may improve because their catheter may move within the blood vessel.

**POSITIVE PRESSURE** - Is pressure greater that zero mmHg. A pressure that is greater than atmospheric pressure. In dialysis, positive pressure is created when the blood pump pushes blood through the pores in the semipermeable membrane. Positive and negative pressure together equal transmembrane pressure. (*See also: Negative Pressure, Transmembrane Pressure, Ultrafiltration*).

**POSTDIALYZER PRESSURE** - See Venous Pressure.

**POSTPUMP ARTERIAL PRESSRUE** - See Predialyzer Pressure.

**POTASSIUM** - A metallic element, and important electrolyte in the human body. Correct levels of potassium are needed for optimal functioning of the body's cells. (*See also: Electrolyte, Hyperkalemia, Hypokalemia*).

**POTTING SOIL** - Polyurethane clay-like material at both ends of the dialyzer that holds the hollow fibers open for blood to flow inside of the fiber.

**PRECIPITATE** - See Scale.

**PREDIALYZER PRESSURE** - Is the positive pressure after the blood pump and before the dialyzer. Predialyzer pressure is also called postpump pressure, or postpump arterial pressure.

**PREPROCESSING** - Means putting a new dialyzer through all the reprocessing steps before it is used for the first time. This process helps remove residual amounts of ETO or other substances used during manufacturing that might cause allergic or hypersensitivity reactions.

**PREPUMP ARTERIAL PRESSURE** - A measurement of the pressure between the patient's arterial needle site and the blood pump. Prepump arterial pressure represents the negative pressure created by the blood pump. Arterial pressure monitoring guards against excessive suction on the vascular access.

**PRESSURE** - A force applied to an object by something that comes in contact with an object. In the human body, blood pressure is the combination of flow or force from the heart, resistance in the blood vessels. In hemodialysis, pressure is the combination of flow from the blood pump and resistance in the dialyzer and extracorporeal circuit.

**PRESSRUE GRADIENT** - See Transmembrane Pressure.

**PRESSURE TESTING** – (Leak testing) Ensures that a dialyzer membrane is intact and no blood loss will occur during the next use. Pressure testing must be a part of the reuse process. (*See also: Reprocessing*).

**PRIMING** - Filling and rinsing the bloodlines and the dialyzer with a solution of normal saline. The priming solution for the dialysate compartments is dialysate. Priming is done before dialysis to remove air, disinfecting chemicals, and some plasticizing chemicals from the extracorporeal circuit and dialysate side of the dialyzer. (*See also: Dialyzer, Disinfectant, Plasticizer*).

**PRIMING VOLUME** - The amount of solution necessary to fill a compartment of the dialyzer before dialysis can begin.

**PRODUCT WATER** - Water that has been forced through a reverse osmosis membrane. (*See also: Reverse Osmosis*).

**PROPORTIONING SYSTEM** - A type of dialysate delivery system. Proportioning systems mix liquid concentrate with specific amounts of treated water to form dialysate and deliver it to the dialyzer. Proportioning systems are available in two types: fixed-ratio pumps and servo-controlled mechanisms. These systems use dual conductivity meters to check the mixed dialysate continuously and to support the system, should one monitor fail. (*See also: Hemodialysis Delivery System*).

**PROTEINURIA** – Means protein in the urine. When kidneys are damaged, protein can leak through the glomeruli into the renal tubules and into the urine. (*See also: Glomerulus, Microalbuminuria*).

**PROXIMAL** - Means nearest the point of attachment, center of the body or point of reference; the opposite of distal.

## PROXIMAL CONVOLUTED TUBULE
– Part of the nephron tubules, which lies between the Bowman's Capsule and the Loop of Henle.

**PRURITUS** - A severe and constant itching. Itching may develop in patients with renal failure due to dry skin or a build-up of calcium phosphate crystals in the skin. Adequate dialysis, good management of calcium phosphorous, limiting bathtub soaking time, and use of some lotions or creams can help reduce itching. Unless pruritus is relieved the patient may become exhausted from lack of sleep.

**PSEUDOANEURYSM** - Is a false aneurysm, a bulging pocket of blood surrounding a fistula or more commonly an ePTFE graft. Pseudoaneurysms can occur if a graft has been repeatedly punctured in the same area. (*See also: aneurysm*).

**PUMP OCCLUSION** - The amount of space between the rollers of the blood pump and the pump housing. The rollers of the blood pump should compress the blood tubing segment against the blood pump house enough to close the lumen completely at that point. Over occlusion produces excess pressure that may crack the tubing causing the pumping segment to rupture. If occlusion is not complete, there will be backflow of blood with each pump stroke. (*See also: Blood Pump Segment*).

**PURE ULTAFILTRATION** - See Isolated Ultrafiltration.

**PURPURA** - Bleeding under the skin, which may be a symptom of heparin overdose or platelet dysfunction. The outward manifestations and laboratory findings of primary and secondary purpura are similar. There is bleeding under the skin, with easy bruising and the development of petechiae . In the acute form there may be bleeding from any of the body orifices, such as hematuria, nosebleed, vaginal bleeding, and bleeding gums. (*See also: Heparin*).

**PYROGEN** - A fever producing substance such as endotoxin – a component of the outer walls of bacteria.

**PYROGENIC REACTION** - Are symptoms caused by pyrogens (such as endotoxins), which may include shills, fever, shaking, hypotension, vomiting, and myalgia. Dialysis patients may have pyrogenic reactions if they are exposed to improperly treated water or an endotoxin-contaminated reprocessed dialyzer. (*See also: Endotoxin*).

# DIALYSIS ACRONYMS
# Q

# Q

**QUALITY ASSURANCE (QA)** - A mechanism or program used by facilities to monitor, evaluate, and improve care. It is based on measuring facilities' quality of care against predetermined standards. (*See also: Clinical Practice Guidelines, Continuous Quality Improvement*).

# DIALYSIS ACRONYMS
# R

# R

**RADIAL ARTERY -** Artery located in the forearm on the thumb side of the wrist.

**RADIAL PULSE –** An artery in the forearm, wrist, and hand; the one usually used for taking the pulse.

**RADIOCEPHALIC FISTULA -** Connects the radial artery and the cephalic vein in the distal forearm to create a vascular access for hemodialysis. This is the most common type of AV fistula.

**REAGENT -** A material that will react in the presence of a certain chemical. Reagent strips are used to make sure all chemical residues are removed from a reprocessed dialyzer or the dialysis delivery system, or test for the presence of blood in dialysate. (*See also: Hemastix*).

**RECIRCULATION -** Occurs when already-dialyzed blood returning to the patient through the venous needle mixes with undialyzed blood entering the arterial needle. Blood entering the dialyzer can become diluted with blood that just left the dialyzer. This occurs as a result of retrograde flow through the vascular access segment between the arterial and venous needle sites. Recirculation greater that 15% is significant, and reduces hemodialysis adequacy. (*See also: Hemodialysis Adequacy, Retrograde*).

**RECOMBINANT** - Means cloned. A recombinant substance such as EPOGEN has been developed by genetic engineering techniques. (*See also: EPOGEN*).

**REJECTION** - Occurs when the immune system of a transplant patient attacks the transplanted organ because it is foreign to the body. The risk of rejection is reduced by matching the patient's blood type and tissue type the organ the body is less likely to recognize the organ as foreign, and by using immunosuppressant drugs to reduce the body's immune response to the transplanted organ.

**REJECT WATER** - The waste or reject stream that is sent to the drain along with the solutes removed by the reverse osmosis.

**RENAL FAILURE** - See acute renal failure, chronic renal failure.

**RENAL NEUROPATHY** – Disease of the nerves caused by chronic renal failure or uremia, causing symptoms such as loss of sensation (or painful sensation) in the hands or feet, muscle weakness, impaired reflexes.

**RENAL OSTEODYSTROPHY** - Generalized pathological changes in bone with resemblance to Osteitis Fibrosa Cystica, osteomalacia, and osteoporosis. These changes are associated with renal failure. The serum phosphorous is elevated, calcium is low or normal, and there is increased parathyroid gland activity.

**RENIN -** An enzyme produced by the kidney to control blood pressure. Renin splits angiostensinogen to form a pressor substance angiostensin I, which is then transformed into angiotensin II, which stimulates vasoconstriction and secretion of aldosterone.

**RENIN-ANGIOSTENSIN-ALDOSTERONE SYSTEM –** Helps control blood pressure in healthy individuals. Renin is an enzyme produced by kidneys during stress. Renin combines with another substance to form angiostensin, a hormone that tightens the blood vessels, raising blood pressure. (*See also: Renin*).

**REPROCESSING -** The process of cleaning and disinfecting dialyzers and, in some cases, bloodlines, to be used on the same patient. Done carefully, reprocessing reduces the cost of dialyzers and offers some benefits to patients. The hazardous chemicals used in reprocessing must be handled with care by staff. A number of regulations and guidelines are in place to protect patients and staff when reprocessed dialyzers are used.

**RESIDUAL BLOOD VOLUME** - The amount of blood remaining in the extracorporeal circuit after termination of hemodialysis treatment.

**RESISTANCE** - Is created by any factor that partially obstructs flow. In dialysis, there is resistance against the flow of blood in the blood vessels or in the extracorporeal circuit. Flow and resistance influence pressure.

**RESISTIVITY** - The measure of the forces that oppose the flow of electricity through a fluid. (*See also: Conductivity*).

**RETROGRADE** - Means against the direction of flow. In a fistula or graft, retrograde flow is toward the anastomosis. The arterial needle may be placed either retrograde or anterograde in the access. (*See also: Anastomosis*).

**REUSE** - The practice of cleaning and sterilizing a used dialyzer that is to be used again by the same patient. (*See also: Reprocessing*).

**REVERSE OSMOSIS** - A membrane separation process for removing solutes from a solution. A reverse osmosis unit is a cartridge containing a water pressure pump and a semipermeable membrane. The RO membrane can remove 90% to 99% of many substances, including bacteria, endotoxin, viruses, salts, particles, and dissolved organics. RO membranes are used to purify or treat the water used for hemodialysis or reprocessing. Because RO membranes are costly and delicate, other filters are used to remove particles in feed water that might damage the RO membrane.

**REVERSE ULTRAFILTRATION** - Moving fluid through the dialyzer membrane from the dialysate compartment into the blood compartment to remove the protein layer that occurs during treatment.

**RINSE BACK** - The process of using saline to flush the patient's blood back into the body after dialysis. The amount of fluid necessary to clear the dialyzer.

**ROLLER PUMP** - Is the most common type of blood pump. A motor turns the roller head, continuously moving blood through the extracorporeal circuit.

# DIALYSIS ACRONYMS
## S

# S

**SAGITTAL PLANE** - A vertical plane through the longitudinal axis of the trunk dividing the body into two portions, right and left.

**SALICYLATE** - A salt of salicylic acid (aspirin).

**SALINE INFUSION LINE** – A line connected to the arterial blood-tubing segment just before the blood pump, so saline can be pulled into the circuit. The saline infusion line allows saline to be given to the patient during dialysis.

**SCALE** – (precipitate) is solid particles that settle out of a solution (i.e., water, dialysate) and can clog pipes or damage components of the water treatment system. Hard water, which contains more minerals and salts, can form scale.

**SECONDARY HYPERPARATHYROIDISM** - The overproduction of parathyroid hormone (PTH) due to renal failure, which can cause bone disease. With too much PTH is the blood, calcium is withdrawn from the bones, making them weak.

**SEDIMENT FILTER** - See filters.

**SEIZURES** - Are involuntary muscle spasms and loss of consciousness. Some patients may have seizures as a dialysis side effect (severe hypotension) or an adverse reaction during dialysis, such as delivery of improperly prepared dialysate.

**SELF-CARE HEMODIALYSIS** - Self-care hemodialysis is a form of in-center hemodialysis in which patients perform most or all of their own care with minimal staff assistance. Self-care patients may set up their own machines, insert needles, take their own vital signs, monitor the treatment, and clean up their station after treatment. Participating in self-care at some level helps the patients regain control of their lives, and helps their rehabilitation.

**SEMIPERMEABLE** – Half-permeable. A membrane that will allow fluids, but not the dissolved substance to pass through it. *(See also: Membrane, Osmosis)*.

**SEMIPERMEABLE MEMBRANE** - A semipermeable membrane is a material with submicroscopic openings or pores. In hemodialysis, the semipermeable membrane's pores allows some substances (such as water) to pass through freely, while keeping other substances (such as red blood cells) from passing through. The size of the pores of the semipermeable membrane is one of the factors that affects the efficiency of the dialysis. Solute particles larger that these pores are retained. Particles small enough to pass through the pores do so at a rate inversely proportional to their size; very small particles pass quicker than larger particles.

**SEPSIS/SEPTICEMIA -** A life threatening infection of the blood caused by bacteria entering the bloodstream. Septicemia is also call bacteremia or sepsis.

**SEQUENTIAL ULTRAFILTRATION -** See Isolated ultrafiltration.

**SERUM -** A serous fluid that moistens the surfaces of serous membranes. The watery portion of blood after coagulation; a fluid found when clotted blood is left standing long enough for the clot to shrink.

**SHUNT -** A bypass. A tube that is inserted into the body. A shunt, or cannula, was the first permanent vascular access for dialysis, developed in 1960 by doctor Belding Scribner and Dr. Wayne Quinton. A Teflon tube was used to connect a flexible length of Silastic tubing to the patient's artery and vein for dialysis, making it possible for patients with chronic renal failure to receive dialysis. Since the shunt was outside the skin, it easily became infected or clotted, and is very rarely used today.

**SODIUM** - An element, and an important electrolyte in the human body. Sodium influences the movement of fluid across the cell membranes between the intracellular and extracellular spaces. Sodium is present in dialysate. Some dialysate delivery systems allow the sodium concentration of the dialysate to be adjusted throughout the treatment, according to a doctor's prescription. The sodium variation has been shown to create more effective fluid removal, as well as better control of blood pressure. Too little sodium in dialysate can cause hemolysis. Too much sodium in dialysate can cause crenation. (*See also: Crenation, Electrolyte, Hemolysis, Hypernatremia, Hyponatremia*).

**SODIUM MODELING** - Refers to tailoring the concentration of sodium in the dialysate to fit the needs of an individual patient, according to the physician's prescription.

**SOLUTE DRAG** - Is the movement of solute molecules along with water through a membrane's tiny pores. Solute drag is also known as convection or convective solute transfer.

**SOLUTES** - Particles dissolved in fluid. Many of the substances that need to be removed from the blood of renal patients (such as urea) are solutes dissolved in the blood. Solute size in measured by molecular weight. Different semipermeable membrane materials are more or less efficient at removing solutes of a certain size. (*See also: Molecular Weight*).

**SOLUTE TRANSFER** – Movement of solutes across the semipermeable membrane. (*See also: Diffusion, Solute Drag*).

**SOLUTION** - A combination of a solvent, or fluid and a solute.

**SPINAL (VERTEBRAL) CAVITY** – Cavity that extends downward from the cranial cavity and is surrounded by bony vertebrae that contains the spinal cord.

**SPHYMOMANOMETER** - An instrument for determining arterial blood pressure indirectly. The two types are aneroid and mercury. (*See also: Blood Pressure*).

**SPORE** - The reproductive form of some bacteria, which are very resistant to heat. Bleach is effective against many spores. The reproductive element, produced sexually or asexually, of one of the lower organisms, such as protozoa, fungi, or algae. (*See also: Bacteria, Disinfectant, Heat Disinfection*).

**STAFF ASSISTED DIALYSIS** –See In-center Hemodialysis.

**STANDARD PRECAUTIONS** – Are infection control procedures that prevent the spread of disease by treating body fluids from all patients as if they could cause infection. Important Standard

Precautions include washing hands, wearing protective clothing, avoiding needle injuries by never cutting or recapping needles, using airway equipment during mouth-to-mouth resuscitation, disposing of infectious waste properly, minimizing the handling of soiled laundry, and cleaning surfaces thoroughly. Standard Precautions combine the major features of Universal Precautions, which reduce the risk of transmitting blood borne pathogens, and Body Substance Isolation, which reduces the risks of transmitting pathogens from moist body fluids and substances.

**STASIS -** A state of equilibrium among opposing forces. A stoppage or diminution of flow, as of blood or another body fluid.

**STORAGE -** A system of conditions under which reprocessed dialyzers are kept until their next use.

**STANDING ORDERS -** Standing orders are orders that stay the same; they are written by the physician to meet the patients' usual treatment needs. The orders should include all aspects of the care of renal patients (i.e., blood flow rate, dialysate flow rate, dialyzer, and dialysate composition).

**STEAL SYNDROME -** Steal syndrome occurs when a fistula or graft "steals" too much blood away from the distal (farthest from the center of body) part of the limb. When the access is in use during dialysis, some of the patients' blood bypasses the hand or foot to pass through the extracorporeal circuit instead. The resulting loss of blood flow or ischemia, can cause tissue damage manifested by coldness, poor function, and even gangrene of the fingertips if it is not addressed promptly. (*See also: Ischemia*).

**STENOSIS -** The narrowing of a blood vessel. Stenosis slows the flow of blood and causes turbulence inside the vessel, setting the stage for more serious complications such as thrombosis. (*See also: Thrombosis*).

**STENTS -** Small expanding metal rings that can be placed inside a fistula or graft or blood vessels that the fistula or graft feeds into (e.g., internal jugular vein) to help keep the lumen from narrowing. Stents are sometimes used to treat stenosis.

**STERILE -** Means completely free of all living organisms (bacteria, viruses, microorganisms).

**STERILE TECHNIQUE -** A series of steps used to maintain a germ-free environment or space. Step in sterile technique include washing hands before touching items in sterile package, touching sterile objects only to other sterile objects, cleaning blood ports or the other patients' skin with disinfectant before inserting a needle, and discarding any sterile supplies in wet, damaged, or torn packages. Peritoneal dialysis exchanges must be done using sterile technique to prevent infection. (*See also: Peritoneal Dialysis*).

**STERILIZATION** - Is the destruction of bacteria with chemicals or heat.

**STREPTOKINASE** - Thrombolytic agent used to help remove thrombi.

**SUBCLAVIAN CATHETER** - A catheter placed in a subclavian vein. According to NKF-DOQI guidelines for vascular access, the subclavian vein is no longer preferred for placement of a temporary or permanent dialysis catheter. Instead, the internal jugular is preferred, because it is less likely to cause central venous stenosis. (*See also: Central Venous Stenosis, Internal Jugular Catheter*).

**SUBCLAVIAN VEIN** - Large vein draining the arm.

**SUBCUTANEOUS** - Means under the fatty layer of skin. Sometimes medications, such as Lidocaine, a local anesthetic are injected subcutaneously.

**SURFACE AREA** - In hemodialysis is the amount of membrane in direct contact with blood and dialysate. A larger surface area (in either hemodialysis or peritoneal dialysis) allows more diffusion. Therefore, large surface area dialyzers normally have more urea clearance. (*See also: Diffusion*).

**SYNTHETIC** - See artificial.

**SYSTEMIC** - Means affecting the entire body. For example, septicemia is a systemic infection.

**SYSTOLIC** - Is the pressure inside the arteries during a heartbeat. It is the top number of a blood pressure reading. (*See also: Diastolic*).

**SYSTOLE** - That part of the heart cycle in which the heart is in contraction. The myocardial fibers are tightening and shortening.

# DIALYSIS ACRONYMS
# T

# T

**TEMPERATURE ALARM -** An alarm that indicates the dialysate temperature is incorrect. Dialysate that is too hot can cause hemolysis. Too cool dialysate can cause patient discomfort and reduce the efficiency of the dialysis.

**TEMPORARY CATHETERS -** A central venous catheter that is used for short-term vascular access, for example, when a permanent access is not mature to use. According to NKF-DOQI guidelines for vascular access, the preferred site for a temporary catheter is the internal jugular (IJ) or femoral vein. Temporary catheters may be stitched or sutured into place. (*See also: Internal Jugular Catheter*).

**THORACIC CAVITY -** The space lying above the diaphragm and enclosed within the walls of the thorax; the space occupied by the thoracic viscera.

**THRILL -** Is the vibration of blood flowing through the patient's fistula or graft. It can be felt by touching a patient's access.

**THROMBECTOMY -** Is a surgery or a chemical treatment (i.e., with a clot dissolving medication) to remove a thrombus or clot.

**THROMBOCYTE** - An old term for blood platelet.

**THROMBOLYSIS** - The process of injecting medication to dissolve a thrombus. Thrombolysis may be followed by surgery.

**THROMBOSIS** - Formation of a thrombus, or blood clot, is the most common cause of access failure. Early thrombosis in a graft or fistula is usually caused by surgical problems with the anastomosis, or by twisting of the vessel or graft.

**THROMBUS** - A clot formed in a blood vessel or a blood passage. A clot may occur when platelets are activated by contact with damaged blood vessel walls, dialyzer materials, or turbulence inside a blood vessel. (*See also: Platelets*).

**TISSUE** - A group or collection of similar cells and their intracellular substance that act together in the performance of a particular function.

**TOTAL CELL VOLUME** - See Fiber Bundle Volume.

**TOTAL PARENTERAL NUTRITION (TPN)** - Is a form of intravenous feeding to provide nutrients to patients who cannot eat or absorb through their gastrointestinal tracts.

Interdialytic parental nutrition (IDPN) is TPN given during dialysis.

**TRANSDUCER PROTECTORS** - Small plastic cones containing filters that prevent blood or fluid from entering the pressure monitors on the dialysis machine. The transducer protectors are connected to the arterial and/or venous pressure monitors, and the monitoring lines are connected to the transducer protectors.

**TRANSMEMBRANE PRESSURE (TMP)** - The pressure across the dialyzer membrane (blood compartment pressure minus dialysate compartment pressure). To keep dialysate fluid from moving into the bloodstream, blood compartment pressure must be equal to or greater that dialysate compartment pressure.

**TRANSPLANT** - To transfer tissue or an organ from one part to another as in grafting or plastic surgery. A piece of tissue or organ used in transplantation.

**TRANSPLANTATION** - The surgical procedure that involves taking an organ or tissue from either a cadaver or a living person and using it to replace a diseased organ or tissue.

**TRANSPORT** - Movement or transfer of substances in a biological system, movement across electrolytes, nutrients, and liquids across cell membranes. Transport may occur actively, passively, or with assistance of a carrier.

**TRANSVERSE PLANE** - Plane that divides the body into a top and bottom portion.

**TREND ANALYSIS** – Review of dialyzer failures and unusual occurrences with equipment and patients in the dialysis environment.

**TRENDELENBERG POSITION** - A body position in which the head is placed at a 45-degree incline, with legs up. This position helps to relieve hypotension. Patients with a suspected air embolism should be placed in the Trendelenburg position on their left side.

**TUBULAR REABSORPTION** - The process by which water and dissolved substances (glomerular filtrate) move from tubules into the blood of peritubular capillaries. Although reabsorption occurs throughout the entire length of the renal tubule, most occurs in the proximal convoluted tubule.

**TWIN CATHETERS** - A form of permanent, silastic, single-lumen, catheters that are used as a permanent vascular access. Each lumen of a twin catheter has a separate subcutaneous tunnel, which may reduce the risk of infection.

# DIALYSIS ACRONYMS
## U

# U

**ULTRADIFFUSION** - Sequential dialysis; separate period of fluid removal and diffusion.

**ULTRAFILTER** - A fine membrane filter that removes very small particles; it is the most effective water treatment component for removing endotoxin. (*See also: Endotoxin*).

**ULTRAFILTRATION** – Filtration caused by a pressure gradient between two sides of a porous (filtering) material. The rate of ultrafiltration depends on the transmembrane pressure (TMP) and the characteristics of the dialyzer. Ultrafiltration also occurs naturally, as in the filtration of plasma at the capillary membrane.

**ULTRAFILTRATION COEFFICIENT (KUF)** - See Coefficient of Ultrafiltration.

**ULTRAFILTRATION RATE (UFR)** - The rate at which fluid moves from the blood into the dialysate through the semipermeable membrane. This rate depends on transmembrane pressure and the characteristics of the semipermeable membrane. The ultrafiltration rate is calculated by dividing the amount of fluid removed by the number of minutes of treatment time. In ultrafiltration control or volumetric machines, dialysate inflow and outflow are exactly balanced through special pumps. (*See also: Transmembrane Pressure*).

**ULTRAFILTRATE** - Fluid removed from the blood.

**ULTRASONOGRAPHY** – A radiologic technique in which deep structures of the body are visualized by recording the reflections (echoes) of ultrasonic waves directed into the tissues.

**ULTRASOUND** – Mechanical radiant energy of a frequency greater than 20,000 Hz; used in medicine in the technique of ultrasonography. (*See also: Ultrasonography*).

**ULTRAVIOLET (UV) LIGHT** - A form of invisible radiation that can destroy microorganisms by altering their DNA (genetic material) so they cannot multiply. Some microorganisms are more sensitive than others to the effects of UV light. Ultraviolet light uses a mercury vapor lamp that emits light at a specific wavelength, housed inside a quartz sleeve. Feed water flows over the quartz sleeve. Feed water flows over the quartz material and is exposed to the UV light. (*See also: Feed Water, Microorganisms*).

**UNIVERSAL PRECATUIONS** - See Standard Precautions.

**UREA** - The chief nitrogenous component of urine. The end product of protein metabolism. The diamide of carbonic acid, a crystalline solid having the formula $CH_4N_2O$; found in blood, lymph and urine.

**UREA KINETIC MODLEING** – A mathematical calculation of the changes in patient's blood urea level during a dialysis treatment. UKM is used to determine whether a patient is receiving adequate dialysis. UKM can also help a physician predict the required time on dialysis, and assess a patient's protein catabolic rate to better meet the patient's dialysis and nutritional needs. The results of UKM are described as Kt/V, in which K is the dialyzer urea clearance in ml/min, t is the length of dialysis in minutes, and V is the volume of blood in which the urea is distributed. NKF-DOQI guidelines for hemodialysis adequacy recommend a minimum delivered Kt/V of 1.2 (prescribed Kt/V of 1.3) for adequate dialysis. BUN levels must be drawn using the slow flow or stop pump technique to ensure accuracy of the Kt/V result. (*See also: Hemodialysis Adequacy*).

**UREA REDUCTION RATIO (URR)** -The simplest method for estimating the delivered dose of dialysis, but it does not provide all the information needed to prescribe a dialysis treatment. BUN levels are measured before and after treatment, and the difference indicates how much urea was removed during dialysis, as a percentage of urea reduction. NKF-DOQI guidelines for hemodialysis adequacy recommend a minimum delivered URR of 65% (prescribed URR of 70%) for adequate dialysis. BUN levels must be drawn using the slow flow or stop pump technique to ensure accuracy of the URR result. (*See also: Hemodialysis Adequacy*).

**UREMIA -** A build-up of wastes in the blood that occurs in the last stage of kidney failure or in patients who are not receiving adequate dialysis, and more dialysis is needed. (*See also: Hemodialysis Adequacy*).

**URETER -** Tubes that connect each kidney to the bladder in order to carry urine out of the body.

**URINE -** An end product of metabolism not needed by the body that is excreted by the kidneys.

# DIALYSIS ACRONYMS
# V

# V

**VASCULAR ACCESS** - A means of repeatedly gaining entry to the patient's blood stream for hemodialysis. A vascular access must permit high enough blood flow rates to ensure effective dialysis. This is accomplished in one of three ways: by surgically connecting a patient's artery and vein to form an arteriovenous fistula, by connecting a patient's artery and vein with a piece of artificial vein (a graft), or by using a plastic tube, or catheter. The vascular access is the patient's lifeline; great care must be taken to protect it through good needle insertion technique and needle site rotation.

**VASOCONSTRICTION** - The decrease in the caliber of blood vessels or narrowing of the blood vessels.

**VASODIALTATION** - Dilation or widening of the blood vessels, small arteries and arterioles.

**VENIPUNCTURE** - Inserting a needle into a blood vessel. Skilled and gentle venipuncture prolongs the life of a patient's access, and enhances patient comfort. Proper venipuncture also helps ensure that the patient will receive a good dialysis treatment. It is also important to rotate venipuncture sites to avoid causing aneurysms or pseudoaneurysms to form the in patient's access. (*See also: Aneurysms, Pseudoaneurysms*).

**VENOUS HYPERTENSION -** A condition caused by stenosis where the venous pressure equalizes with arterial pressure causing swelling in the hand especially the thumb.

**VENOUS PRESSURE -** The measurement of the extracorporeal blood circuit pressure after the dialyzer and before the blood re-enters the patient's body. It may also be called post dialyzer pressure.

**VENOUS PRESSURE HIGH/LOW ALARM -** An alarm that monitors pressure from the monitoring site (venous chamber) to the patient's venous puncture site.

**VENTRAL CAVITY -** The cavity that is located toward the front part of the body. It is divided by the diaphragm into the upper thoracic cavity and the lower abdominopelvic cavity.

**VIRUSES -** Microorganisms that must obtain energy and food from other living cells. Many human diseases, such as the common cold, measles, polio, and HIV, are caused by viruses. Although extremely small, viruses are too large to cross an intact dialyzer membrane. However, if the membrane is damaged, any viruses contained in the dialysis water could contaminate the patient's blood. Viruses can be destroyed by various chemicals.

**VOLUMETRIC -** Means volume-measuring. Most dialysate delivery systems use volumetric fluid-balancing systems that compare the volume of dialysate entering and leaving the dialyzer. With volumetric control, the delivery system can be programmed to remove precisely the prescribed amount of fluid, delivering an exact prescription for ultrafiltration.

# DIALYSIS ACRONYMS
# W

# W

**WATER SOFTENER -** A component used in the water treatment system to reduce the concentration of calcium and magnesium in water that form scale. Water softeners work by a process of ion exchange. Ions of calcium and magnesium are removed from the water by a bed of electrically charged resin beads and traded for sodium ions, which form sodium chloride.

# DIALYSIS ACRONYMS
# X

# X

**XYLOCAINE** - The trade name for Lidocaine Hydrochloride.

# Essential Terms of Direction and Movement

**Abduction** – Draws away from midline.

**Adduction** – Draws toward the midline.

**Anterior or Ventral** – Situated before or in front of.

**Distal** – Farther from the root.

**Dorsal or Posterior** – Toward the rear, back; also back of hand and top of foot.

**Extension** – Straightening.

**External** – Outside.

**Frontal or Coronal** – Vertical; at right angles to sagittal; divides body into anterior and posterior parts.

**Horizontal** – At right angles to vertical.

**Inferior** – Lower, farther from crown of head.

**Internal** – Inside.

**Inverted** – Turned inward.

**Lateral** – Farther from the midline.

**Longitudinal** – Refers to long axis.

**Medial** – Nearer to midline.

**Median** – Midway, being in the middle.

**Midline** – Divides body into right and left side.

**Palmar** – Palm side of the hand.

**Plantar** – Sole side of the foot.

**Posterior or Dorsal** – Rear or back.

**Prone** – Forearm and hand turned palm side down.

**Proximal** – Nearer to limb root.

**Sagittal** – Vertical plane or section dividing body into right and left portions.

**Superficial** – Nearer to surface.

**Superior** – Upper, nearer to crown of head.

**Supine** – Forearm and hand turned palm side up.

**Ventral or Anterior** – Situated before or in front of.

**Vertical** – Refers to long axis in erect position.

# Related Web Sites

Dialysis Online! Message Boards:
www.be.net/~brumley/renal/index/html

Early Renal (Disease) Handbook
www.nephron.com/fkgframeset.html

Early Kidney Disease website for patients:
www.kidneydirections.com
by Baxter healthcare Corporation

E-Neph (website for journal Dialysis and Transplantation):
www.eneph.com

Polycystic kidney disease:
www.pkdcure.org

Health Care Financing Administration (HCFA):
www.hcfa.gov

Hypertension, Dialysis, and Clinical Nephrology (HDCN):
www.medtext.com/bdcn.htm

National Institute of Diabetes & Digestive & Kidney Disease (NIDDK):
www.niddk.nih.gov

National Transplant Assistance Fund (NTAF):
www.transplantfund.org

The Nephron Information Center:
www.nephron.com

Renalnet:
www.renalnet.com

Renal Rehabilitation Life Option Council:
www.lifeoptions.org

TransWeb (transplantation and donation information):
www.transweb.org

United Network for Organ Sharing (UNOS):
www.unos.org

U.S. Renal Data System (USRDS):
www.med.umich.edu/usrds

**Diabetes:**

American Diabetes Association:
www.diabetes.com

American Diabetes Association (basic article on kidney disease and diabetes):
http://www.diabetes.org/ada/c70f.asp

DiabeticNet:
http://www.diabeticnet.com/articles/kidney.htm

# Suggestions

If you have suggestions for this book please send them to:

**Medical West Publishing**
P.O. Box 22
West Covina, CA 91793
USA

Or you can e-mail us at:

mwp@medicalwestpublishing.net

Other books by Oscar M Cairoli:

- **Memory Bank for Hemodialysis** – 1982 and 1986

- **The Dialysis Handbook for Technicians and Nurses** – 2003 and 2012

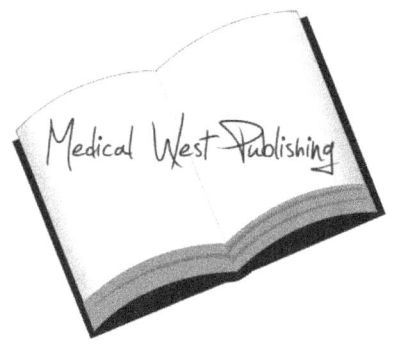

# Medical West Publishing

medicalwestpublishing.net

*P.O. Box 22*
*West Covina, California*
*USA*
*91793*

## Oscar M Cairoli, BSN, MA, RN, PHN

The author has over 35 years in the field of Nephrology/Dialysis. He has a BSN and Masters in Management and a Public Health Certification from the state of California. He has written multiple papers regarding dialysis, as done presentations all over the country.

www.ingramcontent.com/pod-product-compliance
Lightning Source LLC
Chambersburg PA
CBHW071524180526
45171CB00002B/366